DELEUZE AND GUATTARI'S
ANTI-OEDIPUS

Anti-Oedipus is one of the most important texts in philosophy to have appeared in the last thirty years. The first collaborative work of Gilles Deleuze and Félix Guattari, it presents a brilliant and devastating critique of the Freudian Oedipus complex by condemning it as a reactionary, guilt-inducing product of capitalist institutions. A truly remarkable and vastly complicated text, *Anti-Oedipus* revolutionized poststructuralism and Continental philosophy.

In *Deleuze and Guattari's* Anti-Oedipus: *Introduction to schizoanalysis* Eugene W. Holland provides a comprehensive yet accessible guide to this complex and notoriously difficult text. He investigates the manner in which Deleuze and Guattari negotiate the interactions between the three main materialist thinkers of modernity, Freud, Marx, and Nietzsche, and lucidly examines the role of schizoanalysis in Deleuze and Guattari's radical materialist psychiatry.

An indispensable guide to *Anti-Oedipus*, this book is a perfect introduction to the early thought of Deleuze and Guattari, celebrating not only the importance and rigor of their work but highlighting its lasting implications for the continuing debates on Marxism, environmentalism and feminism.

Eugene W. Holland is Associate Professor of French and Comparative Literature at the Ohio State University.

DELEUZE AND GUATTARI'S
GUATTARI'S
ANTI-OEDIPUS

Introduction to schizoanalysis

Eugene W. Holland

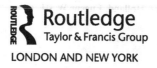

Routledge
Taylor & Francis Group

LONDON AND NEW YORK

First published 1999
by Routledge

Published 2014 by Routledge
2 Park Square, Milton Park, Abingdon, Oxon OX14 4RN

Simultaneously published in the USA and Canada by Routledge
605 Third Avenue, New York, NY, 10017, USA

Routledge is an imprint of the Taylor & Francis Group, an informa business

©1999 Eugene W. Holland

Typeset in Times by Routledge

British Library Cataloguing in Publication Data
A catalogue record for this book is available from the British Library

Library of Congress Cataloging in Publication Data
Holland, Eugene W.
Deleuze and Guattari's Anti-Oedipus : introduction to schizoanalysis /
Eugene W. Holland
p. cm.
Includes bibliographical references and index
1. Social psychiatry. 2. Psychoanalysis—Social aspects.
3. Oedipus complex—Social aspects. 4. Capitalism.
5. Schizophrenia—Social aspects. I. Guattari, Félix.
II. Holland, Eugene W. III. Title.
RC455.D42213   1999
194—dc21   CIP

ISBN 13: 978-0-415-11319-9 (pbk)
ISBN 13: 978-0-415-11318-2 (hbk)

CONTENTS

PREFACE

This book is intended as an introduction to reading Deleuze and Guattari's *Anti-Oedipus*, not as a substitute for it. If this introduction encourages people to read – or re-read – the original, its aim will have been fulfilled; anyone who reads this book will be well prepared to read and enjoy *Anti-Oedipus* itself. Anyone who reads this book instead of the original, however, will be making a sorry mistake, for they will miss the chance to encounter first-hand one of the most fascinating and compelling experiments in recent French thought, an experiment that Deleuze and Guattari called "schizo-analysis."

The experiment is both intricate and far-reaching, and the resulting book is quite difficult – albeit for specific reasons that I will explain in what follows. Indeed, those well-versed in Deleuze and Guattari's works appear to have had as much difficulty with it as have those for whom *Anti-Oedipus* represents the initial encounter with Deleuze and Guattari: despite the title's notoriety, little sustained scholarly attention has been focused on the book in its own right. Experienced readers of Deleuze and Guattari may stand to benefit as much as do neophytes, then, from an introduction to schizoanalysis.

Anti-Oedipus is the first-fruit of a remarkable (and long-lasting) collaboration between philosopher Gilles Deleuze and anti-psychiatrist Félix Guattari. Guattari can be considered the rough equivalent in France of R. D. Laing or David Cooper in England, Thomas Szaz or Ernest Becker in the United States – except that Guattari, in addition to being a leading theoretician of the innovative La Borde psychiatric clinic, was also a militant political activist who always sought to link his (anti-)psychiatric reforms and theorization to working-class and community-based revolutionary politics. Gilles Deleuze, meanwhile, was an apparently quite strictly academic philosopher, best-known initially for studies of the Western tradition's maverick philosophers (such as Bergson and Spinoza, with Kant being the important exception), until his major contributions to French post-structuralism and its "philosophies of difference" appeared in the late 1960s. Indeed, it may be that the events of 1968 brought these two otherwise quite unlikely collaborators together in a way that would be unthinkable outside the context of that tumultuous and fertile moment, and that their thought-experiment was conducted in an effort to respond to it. But the fruit of that collaboration is, in any case, quite unlike either the Anglo-American anti-psychiatry, to which Guattari's work bears certain affinities, or the Frankfurt School's synthesis of Marx and Freud (particularly the "negative dialectics" of Theodor Adorno), to which Deleuze's poststructuralist philosophy of difference could usefully be compared. Without attempting the impossible (and in any case pointless) task of trying to determine exactly what in *Anti-Oedipus* comes from the one and what from the other, it could be said that while Deleuze dramatically deepens Guattari's anti-psychiatric stance by grounding it in an alternative philosophical tradition featuring Nietzsche, Spinoza, and Bergson rather than Plato, Descartes, and Hegel, Guattari at the same time dramatically sharpens Deleuze's philosophical perspective by bringing it into contact with theoretical and institutional struggles in French psychoanalysis and psychiatry, and with the political turmoil surrounding students' and workers' movements in France and throughout Europe (particularly Italy). As much because of the moment in which it emerged as because of the quite disparate figures that were its authors, schizoanalysis is, to say the least, a quite extraordinary venture in experimental thinking and writing.

My first book *Baudelaire and Schizoanalysis* aimed to show what schizoanalysis can contribute to the field of literary and cultural history. It combined intensive reading of Baudelaire's poetic texts and essays with extensive socio-historical contextualization of the emergence of modernism in mid-nineteenth-century France. The present book, in some ways a sequel to the first, is both less ambitious and more so: it is not as specialized and detailed, but at the same time it aims to be both comprehensive and accessible in its presentation of schizoanalysis. Comprehensive yet accessible: that is no easily accomplished task. For *Anti-Oedipus* is an extremely complicated work that draws on a prodigious range of sources, not all of which can be treated adequately in a book of this scope. Indeed, to follow up all or even most of Deleuze and Guattari's references to art and literature, anthropology and ethnography, economics, psychology, physics, aesthetics, biology, philosophy, mathematics, and so on, would require a book several times the size of *Anti-Oedipus* itself. So a short introduction to schizoanalysis, such as this is, will necessarily be very selective, leaving out much that could have been included.

For the purposes of this introduction, I consider schizoanalysis to draw principally on the three great materialists of the last century – Freud, Marx, and Nietzsche – and it is on schizoanalysis as a revolutionary "materialist psychiatry" that I concentrate here. I must thereby forgo treating in detail Deleuze and Guattari's debts to Spinoza and Bergson, for example, or to chaos theory and molecular biology. The former are explained with admirable lucidity by Michael Hardt (in *Gilles Deleuze: an Apprenticeship in Philosophy*), while the latter figure significantly in Brian Massumi's extraordinary book

(*A User's Guide to Capitalism and Schizophrenia*). This introduction to schizoanalysis lies squarely in-between these two equally valuable but quite different works: Hardt's book examines the relation of Deleuze's early work to Bergson, Spinoza, and Nietzsche; later encounters with Guattari, Marx, and Freud lie beyond its scope. Massumi, meanwhile, treats the two volumes of *Capitalism and Schizophrenia* as a whole, but tends to emphasize the topics and perspectives of the second volume, *A Thousand Plateaus*, over those of *Anti-Oedipus*. (Relatively little mention is made of Freud and Lacan, for example, in either *A Thousand Plateaus* or Massumi's *User's Guide*, whereas they are fundamental reference-points, obviously, for *Anti-Oedipus*.)

At the same time, it must be said that the second volume of *Capitalism and Schizophrenia* has proven more durable or popular than the first. In one sense it is the more accessible: whereas *Anti-Oedipus* mounts one long complex argument (appearances to the contrary notwithstanding), *A Thousand Plateaus* operates on many fronts at once; one really can, as the authors recommend, explore any of the plateaus in its own right, and pick and choose which to read and which to skim or skip over. More telling, however, is the more cautious and sober tone of the second volume; the revolutionary enthusiasm of *Anti-Oedipus* appears to be dampened if not silenced in *A Thousand Plateaus*. And this for determinate historical reasons, no doubt: as I argued in *Baudelaire and Schizoanalysis*, the period succeeding the revolutionary outburst of 1968 in France – much like the period succeeding the short-lived revolution of 1848, two economic long-waves before – is a time of retrenchment. *Anti-Oedipus* (1972) was published in the afterglow of the events of May 1968, before the first "oil shock" of 1974 put an end to hopes for widespread social transformation in France (and elsewhere); *A Thousand Plateaus* (1980) – published in the thick of the oil crisis (1974–81) – is both less engaged with pressing socio-historical events and far richer and broader in scope.

Anti-Oedipus should therefore be understood partly as an inspiration and a reflection of May 1968: because of its revolutionary enthusiasm, to be sure, and its rationale for the kind of de-centralized, small-scale, and impro-visational "micro-political" struggle that took place in Paris and then throughout France in the spring of that year; but also because of its critique of party power-structures (and implicitly, therefore, of the French Communist Party and its betrayal of students and workers in siding with the Gaullist forces of law and order). Yet the book should also be understood, as Michel Foucault insists in his 1977 Preface to the English edition, in a less time-bound fashion as an ethics or politics of what he calls "anti-fascism," by which he means opposition to "not only historical fascism...but also the fascism in us all, in our heads and in our everyday behavior, the fascism that causes us to love power, to desire the very thing that dominates and exploits us" (xiii). In this respect, it is precisely because we have passed from a period of revolutionary enthusiasm for social change to one of retrenchment and quiescence that the lessons of *Anti-Oedipus* remain so vitally important:

historically short-sighted as it may be so to do, people are all the more likely to become enamored of power and everyday fascism when these forces seem to have won the day and to represent the only game in town. Whether swimming against or with the historical tide, schizoanalysis carries the fight against fascism and power well beyond battles with the French Communist Party or with the state, extending it into ethical, cultural, familial, personal, and libidinal domains, in addition to the economic and the political. And anyway, this period of quiescence, too, will pass.

As Foucault's allusion to the schizoanalytic diagnosis of "fascism in our heads" suggests, Deleuze and Guattari work at the intersection of politics and psychiatry, not to mention aesthetics, economics, semiotics, and many other fields. Fascism is not just a political or historical term, for example, but also a psychological one – and much the same could be said conversely of terms like schizophrenia and paranoia, which become political and historical terms rather than merely psychological ones. *Anti-Oedipus* is in this sense an exercise in the invention or re-invention of concepts (which Deleuze and Guattari insist in their last collaborative work, *What Is Philosophy?*, is the very purpose of philosophy). The propensity to create new concepts and radically adapt and transfigure old ones undoubtedly contributes to the terminological difficulties of reading their work. (Philip Goodchild has even included a glossary of terms in his survey, *Deleuze and Guattari: an Introduction to the Politics of Desire*.) Here, I have dropped some specialized terms and retain only the more important ones, such as *desiring-machines, desiring-production, body-without-organs, deterritorialization*, and *axiomatization*; even when they are unwieldy, they play a crucial role in the argument, as we shall see. In every case, I have tried to show how the specialized terms or neologisms are derived from or relate to existing and better-known terminology. But I have also provided, in the notes to the text, extensive quotations from the original, so as to let Deleuze and Guattari speak for themselves – and as a way of leading readers back to *Anti-Oedipus* itself. Viking Penguin has kindly granted its permission for such extensive quotation.

Much misunderstanding has arisen about Deleuze and Guattari's particular use of the term "schizophrenia" in particular. Borrowed initially from psychiatry, the term will in their hands designate one pole of the economic, cultural, and libidinal dynamics of capital (the other pole being designated by the term "paranoia"). To be more precise, Deleuze and Guattari use schizophrenia to refer to a specific mode of psychic and social functioning that is characteristically both produced and repressed by the capitalist economy. In the worst cases – when capitalism is unable to countenance the process of schizophrenia it has itself produced – the result is "madness": schizophrenia as *process* succumbs to a repression that generates "the schizophrenic" as *entity* and the miseries of the psychiatric patient. But in the best cases the process of schizophrenia takes the form of viable social practices and the joys of unbridled, free-form human interaction.

The best concrete illustration of the *process* of schizophrenia I know of is improvisational jazz. Whenever references are made here (as in *Anti-Oedipus*) to schizophrenia as the principle of freedom or the realization of universal history, readers should think of jazz, which represents a fulfillment of the process of schizophrenia, rather than thinking of mental illness, which represents the defeat of that process by the forces of power and repression. In much the same way that we can place a jazz band at one end of a continuum which has a symphony orchestra at the other, we can contrast the game of soccer with the game of (North American) football. Football teams and symphony orchestras share a certain mode of organization and operation: both require an intensive and rigid specialization of roles; in both, order is imposed from above on the group's activity by specially designated members, whether as composer or coach, conductor or quarterback. In soccer and jazz, by contrast, group organization is less rigidly structured, and interaction within the group is more spontaneous and free-form. Soccer players rarely follow set plays; there is no quarterback, and soccer coaches play a relatively minor role. Jazz musicians, likewise, rarely use a score, and continually depart from well-known melodies in their improvised solos: the point is not to slavishly reproduce or "interpret" an existing piece of music, but to produce something new and unique – something unheard-of which nevertheless still "makes sense" to fellow musicians and audience alike. The ideal is to take just enough of what is already known – a melody, a chord-sequence, a harmonic mode or tone-system – as a point of departure for the shared production and enjoyment of what is radically new.

In *The Eighteenth Brumaire of Louis Napoleon* Marx describes bourgeois revolution as an occasion on which real social relations could not live up to the expectations created by its own rhetoric ("liberty, equality, fraternity"), as an occasion on which "the phrase went beyond the content"; and he does so in order to contrast that situation with the revolution to come, where "the content would go beyond the phrase." In a similar way, symphony orchestras can only hope their performances rise to the genius of the composer whose work they are performing: they hope their content lives up to the pre-existing phrase. (Here the past, as Marx put it, weighs like a dead hand upon the living.) In jazz, by contrast, the past enables rather than constrains the present: the improvised performance always exceeds the pre-existing musical composition or structure in complexity, nuance, and originality: the whole point is that the content go beyond the phrase. As an illustration of the process of schizophrenia, then, jazz not only presents to my mind an ideal instance of human relations and interpersonal dynamics but actually suggests a social ideal: the use of accumulated wealth as a basis for the shared production and enjoyment of life in the present rather than the reproduction and reinforcement of power-structures from the past.

Some people may have objections to this analogy between jazz and what Deleuze and Guattari call the process of schizophrenia: it may appear insufficiently political, for example, or may jump too abruptly from the field of aesthetics or everyday life to that of economics or politics, without the requisite intervening mediations. (Deleuze professed "incompetence" about jazz when I suggested the analogy to him.) In the same vein, Deleuze and Guattari admit that there may be objections to what they present under the rubric of schizoanalysis:

> Those who have read us this far [three pages from the end of the book!] will perhaps find many reasons for reproaching us: for believing too much in the pure potentialities of art and even of science; for denying or minimizing the role of classes and class struggle; for militating in favor of an irrationalism of desire; of identifying the revolutionary with the schizo; for falling into familiar, all-too-familiar traps. This would be a bad reading, and we don't know which is better, a bad reading or no reading at all.

Deleuze and Guattari were not concerned to counter possible objections, and neither in this book am I. The aim here is primarily to prevent bad readings of *Anti-Oedipus*. And since it is a difficult enough task simply to present schizoanalysis, I have refrained here from evaluating or critiquing it at the same time. Others have had ample opportunity to do that (usually based on bad readings, sometimes apparently on no reading at all), and there may be occasion for me to do so in a subsequent book, at least as far as French poststructuralism and Marxism are concerned. My purpose for now is thus not to pass judgment, but to enable others to understand, enjoy, and draw their own conclusions from the thought-experiment called schizoanalysis by returning to read or re-read *Anti-Oedipus* for themselves.

This book was begun while on a short leave from the Ohio State University, for which I have my former Chairpersons Charles Williams and Tom Kasulis, and my former Dean G. Michael Riley, to thank. It was completed while I was fortunate to be a Scholar-in-Residence at the Center for Cultural Studies at the University of California, Santa Cruz. I would like to thank its directors, Gail Hershatter and Chris Connery, along with Phil Stevens and Katy Elliott, for helping make my stay there such a stimulating and productive one. I also enjoyed and benefited from conversations with Bob Meister, whom I would like to thank for his insights and suggestions. Most important, as always, are my thanks to Eliza and Lauren for all their support in helping me bring this project to fruition.

Material from *Anti-Oedipus* by Gilles Deleuze and Félix Guattari, translated by Helen Lane, Mark Seem, and Robert Hurley (translation copyright 1977 by Viking Penguin, Inc., English language translation) is used by permission of Viking Penguin, a division of Penguin Putnam, Inc.

Eugene W. Holland
Santa Cruz and Columbus

1

INTRODUCTION

The *Anti-Oedipus* is not easy to read.[1] Anyone accustomed to standard critical discourse – to the careful presentation and justification of categories, the patient edification of conceptual frameworks, the desire to put everything in a clearly-defined place and have the final word – will probably find the shape and tenor of Deleuze and Guattari's discourse unsettling and perplexing, if not downright maddening. The book starts by describing in minute and sensory details the workings of what it calls "desiring-machines," as if their existence or very definition could be taken for granted, and ends up feigning incompetence.[2] Allusions to modern theoretical mathematics co-exist with references to "primitive" mythology: the semiology of the genetic code stands side-by-side with the differential calculus of finance capital. Bizarre terms such as the "body-without-organs" and images like "flying bricks" suddenly appear without explanation and often equally quickly disappear for no apparent reason. No wonder one of the team of English translators described the book as an "experiment in delirium" (xviii). But it is "a carefully constructed and executed experiment" (xviii), as they go on to say; there is a method to the madness. Understanding why the book was written the way it was can be a first step in better understanding how to read it.

Deleuze and Guattari were of course not alone in developing unorthodox "writing styles" or discursive strategies in the wake of structuralism in France. Derrida, for one, used parody, sarcasm, crossed-out words, and neologisms to undermine the stability of concepts in philosophical discourse and denounce the vain hope of fixing firm boundaries between concepts and metaphors.[3] Perhaps even more than Derrida's own influential texts, *Anti-Oedipus* plays wildly with the permeability of boundaries between concept and metaphor. And yet Deleuze and Guattari insist that schizoanalytic categories such as "desiring-machines" are not to be dismissed as "mere" metaphors.[4] As wild or as fanciful as it may at first seem, the term "desiring-machines" functions to connect the Freudian concept of libido with the Marxian concept of labor-power, and this conceptual connection, rigorously pursued throughout *Anti-Oedipus*, lies at the heart of schizoanalysis.

1

Equally influential but closer to the concerns of *Anti-Oedipus* was the unorthodox discursive style of Lacan, developed initially for training psycho-analysts. Since fixed meaning is a neurotic delusion according to Lacan, discourse is to be deployed in such a way as to circumvent or belie determinate meaning and demonstrate instead the volatile dynamics of the unconscious in language itself. In a similar way, although with a very different conception of the unconscious, Deleuze and Guattari set out to write *Anti-Oedipus* in accordance with the dynamics of unconscious thought, in an attempt to reproduce as much as possible the dynamics of what they call (drawing on Melanie Klein and Lacan) the process of *schizophrenia*. The book not only takes psychosis rather than neurosis as its point of departure, and constructs a model of the psyche based on psychotic rather than neurotic dynamics, but adopts a schizophrenic style, appearing almost as if a schizophrenic had written it. But why would they choose to write a book from the perspective of schizophrenia?

It is important first of all to dispel the most common misconception about schizoanalysis, by explaining what Deleuze and Guattari do not mean by "schizophrenia," and why they claim never to have seen a schizophrenic (380/456).[5] For schizoanalysis, schizophrenia is not the disease or mental disturbance characterizing or defining schizophrenics. Schizophrenics as clinical patients (and "schizophrenia" as a reductive and ill-conceived psych-iatric diagnosis) result, on the contrary, from the incompatibility between the dynamics of schizophrenia unleashed by capitalism and the reigning institutions of capitalist society – including *prima para omnes* the institutions of psychiatry, psychoanalysis, and the nuclear family; hence the sub-title of *Anti-Oedipus*, "Capitalism and Schizophrenia." Schizoanalysis does not romanticize asylum inmates and their often excruciating conditions of exis-tence; it construes schizophrenia in broad socio-historical rather than narrowly psychological terms, as the result of a generalized production of psychosis pervading capitalist society (a process no single psychiatric patient could possibly embody).[6]

Capitalism fosters schizophrenia, in brief, because the quantitative calcu-lations of the market replace meaning and belief-systems as the foundation of society. In a first approximation, then, we could define schizophrenia as a form of "unlimited semiosis" – in the psyche as well as throughout society – that emerges when fixed meanings and beliefs are subverted by the cash nexus under capitalism. Hence a first reason to write *Anti-Oedipus* from the perspective of schizophrenia: schizophrenia constitutes an objective tendency of capitalist society and of its historical development. Every extension of capital – both geographical (imperialism) and psychological (marketing) – entails the simultaneous elimination of extant meanings and beliefs, and hence the extension of schizophrenia: "all that is solid melts into air," as Marx put it. To be sure, a powerful capitalist counter-tendency to schizophrenia exists: Deleuze and Guattari designate it, too, by what was originally a psychological term: *paranoia*. If we understand schizophrenia (in this first approximation) to designate unlimited semiosis, a radically fluid and extemporaneous form of meaning, paranoia by contrast would designate an absolute system of belief where all meaning was permanently fixed and exhaustively defined by a supreme authority, figure-head, or god.[7]

Despite their psychological origins, the terms "paranoia" and "schizophrenia" for Deleuze and Guattari designate effects of the fundamental organizing principles and dynamics of capitalist society. And paranoia represents what is archaic in capitalism, the resuscitation of obsolete, or traditional, belief-centered modes of social organization, whereas schizophrenia designates capitalism's positive potential: freedom, ingenuity, permanent revolution. Hence a second reason to write from the perspective of schizophrenia, even though *Anti-Oedipus* textually embodies both opposing tendencies – paranoia in its inclusion of everything from cell biology to economics, from anthropology to avant-garde poetry, in what appears to be a single all-embracing system; schizophrenia in its ultimate subversion of such systematicity by a highly figurative style of discourse and the use of terms like "desiring-machines" and "body-without-organs" that belie the distinction between concept and metaphor: schizophrenia designates not just an objective tendency of capitalism but the *preferable* objective tendency, in its opposition to the paranoia of tradition and in its potential for radical freedom. The primary aim of schizoanalysis is to take this preferable tendency to the limit, and indeed *push it through the limits*, imposed on it by capitalist paranoia: schizophrenia as revolutionary breakthrough rather than psychological breakdown, as Deleuze and Guattari (following R.D. Laing) put it.[8]

This brings us to a third reason for writing from the perspective, and more specifically in the style, of schizophrenia. *Anti-Oedipus* aims not only to promote a broader understanding of schizophrenia but to promote schizophrenia itself; not merely to reformulate our understanding of desire but to reshape the very form our desires take. The book itself, in other words, was designed to function as a kind of desiring-machine, to program or produce, as well as to model or comprehend, desire in schizophrenic form. This gambit has not, in my opinion, worked as well as it might; despite being a best-seller among works of recent philosophy, the book has not really had the impact it deserves. So I have opted not to attempt to reproduce the "stylistic" schizophrenia of *Anti-Oedipus* in this book, but to concentrate instead on the broader outlines of schizoanalysis itself; my aim above all is to make *Anti-Oedipus* as useful as possible, not to remain faithful to what may have been one of the animating intentions of the authors. Still, the book is a machine; and about a machine one asks not what it might mean but *what it can do* and *how it works*.

How it works (1): the materialisms of Freud, Marx, and Nietzsche

Like schizophrenic desire, *Anti-Oedipus* works by making certain connections – between libido and labor-power, most fundamentally – and by
rejecting others – the clinical definition of "schizophrenia," for example, but
also the psychoanalytic definition of desire as "lack." The result is a thor-
ough reconfiguration of the social landscape invested by desire. Crucially for
Deleuze and Guattari, the processes of connection and rejection always
precede the moment of reconfiguration, when stock is taken of the work
that has been performed and a new configuration becomes recognizable. Yet
using this view of desire as an organizing principle for a book such as *Anti-
Oedipus* presents most readers with difficulties: they often find themselves
starting *in media res*, immersed in a plethora of details, and may finally
come to an understanding of the point of the argument only when it is
reaching its conclusion.

As a first approximation, we can say that the machinery of *Anti-Oedipus*
is set up to produce schizoanalysis from the ruins or remnants of psychoanalysis.[9] The book is basically transformative: it produces concepts –
desiring-machines, schizophrenia, and others – that are themselves productive, that alter our understanding of desire and of society, and do so while
(hopefully) transforming our desires themselves and society with them.
Although the range of raw materials used in this transformative enterprise is
staggering, the three great materialisms formulated at the end of the last
century – those of Marx, Nietzsche, and Freud – constitute major points of
departure.[10] Obviously, and as the title makes clear, Freudian psychoanalysis
is one point of departure and the principal object of critique: schizoanalysis,
drawing substantially on Marx, transforms psychoanalysis so as to include
the full scope of social and historical factors in explanations of behavior and
cognition. Yet psychoanalysis is not rejected wholesale[11]: in the process of
transforming psychoanalysis, schizoanalysis – drawing now on Freud and
especially Lacan – transforms historical materialism so as to include the full
scope of libidinal and semiotic factors in its explanations of social structure
and development. Ultimately, though perhaps least obviously, both structural psychoanalysis and historical materialism are transformed by
Nietzsche's critique of asceticism and his transvaluation of difference, which
inform both the libidinal and the social economies mapped by schizoanalysis. Of course, Deleuze and Guattari are not the first to attempt to
negotiate or forge relations among Freud, Marx, Nietzsche, in one combination or another. But their strategy and conclusions are quite distinctive, and
bear comparison with those of others.

The best-known attempts to combine insights from Marx and Freud are
probably those of Herbert Marcuse, in *Eros and Civilization*, and Wilhelm
Reich, in *The Function of the Orgasm* – both of which are cited as precursors
in *Anti-Oedipus*. Marcuse's "Philosophical Inquiry into Freud" (as per his

subtitle) in effect grafts socio-historical notions of surplus-production (derived from Marx) and of domination (derived from Weber) onto Freud's model of repression, thereby transforming his view of the history of repression (expressed most succinctly in *Civilization and its Discontents*). Marcuse targets the relation between the pleasure principle and the reality principle, as Freud construes it: although he grants that pleasure's demand for immediate gratification must be tempered by the reality principle in the face of scarcity, Marcuse also insists that scarcity is always socially managed, and indeed distributed unevenly, in the service of social domination. Repression of pleasure by reality is supplemented by a *surplus-repression* sustaining class hierarchies; the reality principle succumbs to the *performance principle*. Gradual rationalization of the performance principle (largely the historical contribution of the bourgeoisie) has finally culminated in the conquest of scarcity, with the result that the very rationality of the performance principle has now become irrational. Marcuse therefore calls for a new, non-performative, re-integration of the pleasure and reality principles, free from the distortions of class domination.

While Deleuze and Guattari agree that Freud must be historicized, they disagree on the status of scarcity: according to schizoanalysis, scarcity is not merely socially managed, but is socially fabricated in order to found and secure social organization in various forms. Following Bataille, Deleuze and Guattari insist that societies have always produced a surplus, no matter how dire the circumstances may have appeared and however minimal that surplus may have been: social organization revolves around the determination of how and by whom that surplus will be expended or distributed. Scarcity never had to be overcome by the development of productive forces, since it was already a fabrication from the start: the performance principle could not have become irrational when productive forces became sufficient, for it was never rational to begin with. Historicizing Freud and foregrounding the social management of imposed scarcity are essential for schizoanalysis, but not in terms of the rational or irrational synthesis of pleasure and reality.

In one respect, though, Marcuse's identification of the social management of scarcity and its implications for the relation of pleasure and reality has a salutary result: since repression is seen to vary historically according to social organization, Freud's Oedipus complex and the myth of the "primal horde" and original patricide have, according to Marcuse, only "symbolic" rather than truly anthropological or historical value.[12] Indeed, the Oedipus complex appears only sporadically in *Eros and Civilization*. Nevertheless, it serves Marcuse as a model for social authority, oppression and repression. Oppressive–repressive authority first extends outward from family to society, from father to chief, priest, or boss, in Marcuse's mythical–historical schema, only to be eclipsed by the overwhelming and all-encompassing power of rationalized social authority (in post-Enlightenment bourgeois society). But this schema reverses the real direction of determination, according to Deleuze and Guattari: for schizoanalysis, social oppression–repression in society at large is always primary with respect to psychic repression in the individual. Moreover, the form of social oppression determines the form of psychic repression, and since the former varies historically (as Marcuse also insists), the latter does not remain constant, and thus does not always take the form of the Oedipus complex. Taking the Oedipus as the model – even only as a "symbolic" model – for repression ends up thwarting Marcuse's own effort to historicize Freudian theory.[13]

On this count, Reich's position is categorical: psychic repression depends on social oppression. That is why Deleuze and Guattari consider him the "true founder of a materialist psychiatry": "Reich was the first to raise the problem of the relationship between desire and the social field (and went further than Marcuse)" (118/141). In particular, Reich raised the problem of fascism in terms of how it was in fact desired by the masses, rather than as a matter of ideology or deception; for "[according to Reich] the masses were not deceived, they desired fascism, and that is what has to be explained" (257/306).[14] Any explanation that grants psychic repression even an autonomy from, much less a precedence over, social oppression–repression risks becoming an apology for the latter.[15]

It is not just the explanatory precedence of social oppression over psychic repression that Deleuze and Guattari commend in Reich, but the latter's own critique of Freud for betraying his discovery of libido or sexuality and the repression of sexuality. Schizoanalysis has its own understanding of what it meant for Freud to forsake his most important discoveries, as we shall see in a moment, but for the most part they agree with Reich's analysis. Positing free-floating anxiety as the cause of sexual repression rather than its result, as Freud came to do, absolves social oppression–repression of any liability. In the same vein, they agree that when Freud translates sexuality into *Eros* and pairs it with *Thanatos*, the primacy of sexuality is lost and the outlook and practice of psychoanalysis become morbid:

> As Reich says, when psychoanalysis begins to speak of Eros, the whole world breathed a sigh of relief: one knew what this meant, and that everything was going to unfold within a mortified life, since Thanatos was now the partner of Eros...
>
> (332/397)

Indeed, Deleuze and Guattari will take Reich's critique one step further, by showing that psychoanalysis did not somehow invent Thanatos or the death instinct; rather it uncritically reproduces in the guise of a psychological instinct what is in fact the product of specific socio-historical circumstances. Here, as with Marcuse, Reich's historicization of psychoanalysis did not go quite far enough, and schizoanalysis will show how death becomes an instinct in the course of historical developments leading up to the contemporary society that Freud's theory reflects.[16]

Yet even though Reich correctly posed the question of sexual repression in relation to social oppression, he was ultimately unable to answer it successfully, according to Deleuze and Guattari. He got the dependence of psychic repression on social oppression–repression right, but misunderstood the nature of the relation between the two. For Reich believes that social relations are governed by a sufficient rationality, while psychology is determined – and indeed distorted – by ideology. The role of an un-reconstructed Marxism for Reich is to understand and further the revolutionary historical movement of increasing productivity, rationality, and potential freedom in the "objective" sphere of society at large, while psychoanalysis is constrained to explain the neurotic inhibitions and irrationalities of the "subjective" private sphere. For schizoanalysis, by contrast, Marxism needs revision to account better for subjectivity, just as psychoanalysis needs revision to account better for the varying circumstances of society and history. Furthermore, the distinction between public and private spheres is not real, but is a misleading appearance peculiar to capitalism: desire, Deleuze and Guattari insist, is part of the infrastructure.

> If Reich, at the very moment he raised the most profound of questions – "Why did the masses desire fascism?" – was content to answer by invoking the ideological, the subjective, the irrational... and the inhibited, it was because he remained the prisoner of derived concepts that made him fall short of the materialist psychiatry he dreamed of, that prevented him from seeing how desire was part of the infrastructure, and that confined him in the duality of the objective and the subjective. (Consequently, psychoanalysis was consigned to the analysis of the subjective, as defined by ideology).[17]
>
> (344–5/412–13)

Schizoanalysis thus seems to perform a merger of political economy with what Lyotard (in a book by the same name) called "libidinal economy," and refuses to give either one analytic priority:

> [L]ibidinal economy is no less objective than political economy, and the political no less subjective than the libidinal, even though the two correspond to two modes of different investments of the same reality as social reality.
>
> (345/413)

In principle, Deleuze and Guattari will refuse to separate political and libidinal economy, and will in effect combine them, instead. Yet, at the same time, it is one of their primary objects of investigation, capitalism, that first created and still maintains the split between the two. It is in this sense, again, that psychoanalysis merely reproduces and reinforces the separation of individual from society (much the same being the case in reverse for Marxism), whereas schizoanalysis will strive to overcome it – without completely succeeding. Terms such as "desiring-production," as we shall see in a moment, are invented and deployed so as to link together libido and labor-power and thereby close the gap between psychoanalysis and Marxism; at the same time, the central chapters of *Anti-Oedipus* are divided in a way that reflects and reproduces the distinction between psychic repression (the focus of Chapter Two) and social oppression–repression (the focus of Chapter Three). Yet inasmuch as schizoanalysis succeeds in radically historicizing psychoanalysis, it could not hope or want to remove from its own work all traces of the actual historical situation within capitalism, in any case. The point is not merely to reflect but to expose and critique the social divisions and forms of alienation promulgated by capitalism.

Attempts to combine the insights of Freud and Nietzsche almost inevitably revolve around their shared conclusion that Western society imposes an increasing burden of guilt on humankind, with which Deleuze and Guattari certainly agree. Yet the most developed exploration of this conclusion, that of Norman O. Brown in *Life Against Death*, ultimately favors Freud over Nietzsche – even while drawing on Nietzsche to rewrite Freud and thereby elucidate "the Psychoanalytic Meaning of History" (as per his subtitle); Deleuze and Guattari, by contrast, will favor Nietzsche's socio-political explanations over the psychological accounts of Freud and Brown.

The supposed "progress" of Western civilization entails an endlessly increasing burden of guilt: modern society, Freud and Nietzsche agree, is "neurotic" or "sick," and at the root of the illness, Brown insists, lies the inability to face death. According to Nietzsche, whoever affirms life must thereby affirm death; indeed, only those strong enough to affirm death can truly affirm life. As Brown puts it, the inability to face death amounts to a repression of the death instinct; his rewriting of Freud insists on matching the analysis of the repression of sexuality, or Eros, about which psychoanalysis has had a lot to say, with analysis of the avoidance of death, the repression of the death instinct, or Thanatos, about which it has said all too little.

Humans are historical beings, Brown argues, because unlike other animals they cannot accept death. Due to their prolonged period of intense gratification, dependence, and protection from reality during infancy, human offspring develop exaggerated expectations for gratification, combined with intense hatred of parents who are ultimately unable to provide it, and equally intense guilt over such hatred, in turn. Capable of renouncing neither their expectations nor their parental bonds, emotionally and psychologically

8

dependent on their parents and unable to accept separation from them (which during the formative years would mean death), children become neurotic. The repressed death instinct fuses with the pleasure principle in the repetition compulsion. The "natural" balance between tension and release of tension goes awry, and as anxiety increases, the return of the repressed death instinct fuels an endless search for complete gratification. In effect, the repression of death leaves humans fixated on all the impossible infantile projects they refused to let die in the past, thereby leaving them unable to live in the present and giving motive force to an obsessive orientation toward the future – to restless historical development and eventually to the unavailing "progress" of consumerism and technologism afforded by capitalism.

Brown also invokes Nietzsche in his revision of the Freudian analysis of money. The primary and original function of money, Brown agrees with Nietzsche, is not to facilitate trade but to create and pay debts and thereby both foster and assuage guilt. In archaic society, Brown argues, such debts were owed primarily to the gods, and they were in principle dischargeable. Indeed they *were* discharged periodically, giving rise to and reflecting a finite cyclical view of time, as contrasted with the infinite linear time of modernity.[18] Ironically, it is when the debt comes to be owed primarily to other people rather than to a deity (with the secularization of Protestantism and the emergence of capitalism), that it becomes infinite and impossible to discharge: unlike the gods, no one person or persons can be taken to be responsible for everyone, so all the debt-payments in the world cannot expunge the lasting sense of guilt. Despite or even because of the centrality of money in modern society, the burden of guilt assumes historically unprecedented proportions: no degree of material acquisition, no amount of compulsory work can balance the accounts. Only a complete refusal of the Protestant–capitalist culture of guilt and debt, Brown suggests, will free us from history, understood in this way as a form of neurosis.

As Brown himself makes clear, the stakes in this interpretation of Freud and history are high: he is seeking to replace socio-historical explanations for repression with a psychological one. "We are here at one of the ultimate crossroads in social theory," Brown avers:

> Freud himself (with his Primal Father), as well as Hegel (with his Master) and Nietzsche (with his Master Race) are, like Marx... compelled in the last resort to postulate external domination and its assertion by force in order to explain repression....[But] to take this line is to renounce psychological explanation ("force" being substituted for psychology) and to miss the whole point of the riddle: How can there be an animal which represses itself?[19]

Compulsory labor as the sacrifice of self to an other is no longer to be understood in terms of an external political or economic oppression (Nietzschean domination or Marxian exploitation) and the subsequent internalization of that oppression as self-repression, but rather as the result of infantile separation-anxiety within the family, and the guilt that arises when separation nonetheless inevitably occurs. For "whereas neither the state nor the antinomy of Master and Slave can be granted to be given by nature," Brown wants to suggest, "the institution of the family can."[20]

This is, of course, precisely where Deleuze and Guattari would disagree: the institution of the family cannot be taken for granted.[21] Indeed, much of Chapter Three of *Anti-Oedipus* is devoted to demonstrating how widely the institutions of human reproduction vary historically. Positing a "universal nature of human infancy" to explain why "the slave is somehow in love with his own chains" amounts in Deleuze and Guattari's view to justifying in advance total resignation to any and all forms of social oppression.[22] Their solution will be not to subordinate socio-historical explanation to universalizing psychology, but to propose an apparently paradoxical model of the psyche, as we'll see, wherein the mechanisms that carry out repression at the same time free the human organism from instinctual determination, so that it is the form of social organization that determines whether psychic repression serves social oppression or escapes it. Social organization for Brown (and Freud) does not so much vary historically as simply increase in intensity over time, so his aim is not primarily the reorganization of social relations, but rather what he refers to as a deep-seated "psychological regeneration," the transformation of "historical consciousness...into psychoanalytic consciousness."[23]

Deleuze and Guattari's theoretical differences with Brown, then, boil down to two, one involving their respective readings of Freud, the other their appropriations of Nietzsche. Brown in effect follows the later Freud in abandoning sexuality, as Reich puts it, by reversing the causal relation between repression and anxiety. For Brown, anxiety – and specifically separation-anxiety[24] – causes repression, and the repression of death in particular fuels the repetition-compulsion: we can only hope to end repression (and thence oppression, presumably) by somehow overcoming our infantile fears of separation and death. For Deleuze and Guattari (following Reich), repression causes anxiety, and eliminating social oppression and the kinds of psychic repression that stem from it is the key to reducing anxiety and thereby freeing the human organism from death-inspired and deadening repetition. According to Deleuze, repetition is not in and of itself compulsive: it only becomes so when death gets converted into an instinct. This process resembles Brown's repression of death, but it occurs only under specific historical circumstances, which Deleuze and Guattari spell out in Chapter Three of *Anti-Oedipus*.

It is striking in this connection that, although Brown draws on Nietzsche to rewrite Freud, he almost never mentions the will-to-power. Indeed, there is a sense in which, despite his acute diagnosis and condemnation of asceticism, Brown remains something of an ascetic, for he construes the historical expansion of humans' abilities and sensibilities in exclusively negative terms: as "Faustian restlessness" deriving wholly from morbid infantile fixations and compulsive repetition. Deleuze, however, by placing the concept of will-to-power at the center of his reading of Nietzsche, thereby construes repetition not as compulsion but as variation, innovation, and creation – as the exercise of life-force which naturally aims always at its own continued health and expansion.[25] Brown, in a word, wants to end history as neurosis, so that humankind might "enter that state of Being which was the goal of his Becoming;"[26] for Deleuze and Guattari, Being is a delusion which traps desire in the snare of representation and thereby represses it: their goal is to release desire from Being so it can enter more freely into Becoming. Far from being a neurosis, history for Deleuze and Guattari is the chance that the development of productive forces beyond capitalism and the expansion of will-to-power beyond nihilism will lead to greater freedom rather than enduring servitude. As important as Freud remains for the schizoanalytic endeavor, then, it is Marx and Nietzsche who provide the basis for this appreciation of history, and it is to them that I turn next.

It was Max Weber who insisted that "whoever does not admit that he could not perform the most important parts of his own work without the work that those two [Marx and Nietzsche] have done swindles himself and others."[27] His interest in combining insights of Marx and Nietzsche is perhaps most obvious in *The Protestant Ethic and the Spirit of Capitalism*, where Weber demonstrates how well reformed Christian psychology (one of Nietzsche's favorite targets) suits the dynamics of capitalist surplus-production (Marx's main focus of analysis). But the key Weberian notion of "rationalization" can also be said to derive from both Nietzsche's analysis of modernity as a degraded culture of equivalence in *The Genealogy of Morals* and Marx's analysis of capitalism as an economy of universal equivalence where "all that is solid melts into air...."[28] Such a convergence is perhaps even more evident in Horkheimer and Adorno's *Dialectic of Enlightenment*: while drawing very clearly on Marx and indeed targeting "bourgeois society" as the culmination of the instrumental rationality of domination, they also draw explicitly on Nietzsche and explicitly credit him rather than Marx with being "one of the few after Hegel who recognized the dialectic of enlightenment."[29] It is Georg Lukács, however, who in one important sense comes closest to the schizoanalytic admixture of Nietzsche and Marx, for in translating Weberian rationalization into "reification," he construes it as a direct effect of the capitalist market.[30]

Capitalist society, according to Deleuze and Guattari, is distinct from all others in that it is based on the "cash nexus" of impersonal market relations. Capitalist society, they agree with Horkheimer and Adorno, "is ruled by equivalence [and] makes the dissimilar comparable by reducing it to abstract quantities."[31] Such rendering-equivalent is performed via the market, according to Deleuze and Guattari, by the basic mechanism of the capitalist economy: what they call the process of "axiomatization," which we will examine in more detail in a moment. What distinguishes their view from those of Weber, Horkheimer and Adorno, and especially Lukács, however, is that this fundamental economic process produces two opposing kinds of cultural effects: "decoding" and "recoding". Whereas the others consider rationalization-reification to be mostly or entirely lamentable, Deleuze and Guattari consider axiomatization to be *ambivalent*: it spawns recoding, which is its negative moment as we'll see, but also fosters decoding, which Deleuze and Guattari consider a positive result. By driving a wedge between the economic process of axiomatization and its cultural effects, which are ambivalent, Deleuze and Guattari are able to avoid the more one-sided pessimism of Weber (the "iron cage" of modernity), Horkheimer and Adorno (the totalitarianism of a one-dimensional culture-industry), and Lukács (the nostalgia for pre-market nineteenth-century realism and corresponding condemnation of the market and everything modern in culture).

It might seem surprising that two thinkers as unlike in some respects as Marx and Nietzsche could be conjoined in any of these ways at all. Indeed, one of the striking and most important features of Deleuze and Guattari's work, and something that distinguishes it sharply from virtually all other versions of poststructuralism, is that it brings Marxian and Nietzschean materialisms into contact with one another in a very compelling way. Although Marx and Nietzsche are both acutely critical of contemporary society, their objects of analysis are quite different – psychology and culture for Nietzsche, economics for Marx – and their conclusions are practically opposite: emancipation from capitalism is to be sought through collective social transformation for Marx, while emancipation from nihilism is to be sought through personal self-transformation for Nietzsche. If they nevertheless can be brought together in *Anti-Oedipus*, it is because of their approach rather than their objects or conclusions: both, I would argue, are – in the most general sense of the term – historical materialists.[32] Both, that is to say, take as their starting points the body, on one hand – its productive force, its will-to-power – and the historical expansion of "what the body can do" (in Spinoza's phrase), on the other. Moreover, both see history critically in terms of developing human forces whose further development is hampered by the very structures – of belief, of social organization – that until recently have spurred their development. Capitalism and asceticism have contributed immensely to what human beings can do, but now stand in the way of all that they could do – and must therefore be done away with, superseded.

It may be that what has obscured the shared engagement of Marx and Nietzsche in what I am calling a general historical materialism is not just their opposing means and ends of historical transformation (collective struggle to realize "communism," individual efforts to realize the "overman"), but also the sense that they were addressing different objects or issues, that their analyses didn't intersect or overlap. In one specific historical case, however, Weber has already demonstrated the extent to which the emergence of modern, Protestant asceticism and of full-fledged industrial capitalism coincide, and has therefore implied that the Nietzschean critique of asceticism and the Marxian critique of capitalism may indeed be historically related, at least. Deleuze and Guattari take the development of a general historical materialism one step further, by adding psychoanalysis into the mix as well: it is not just Protestant Christianity in Northern Europe but the nuclear family itself, as the strictly capitalist form of human reproduction, that produces asceticism. With its focus on the dynamics of the nuclear family, psychoanalysis is thus crucial to understanding how ascetic psychology gets produced under, and in turn contributes to, capitalist social organization – even though Freud mistook the capitalist family-form for a universal form of human reproduction, and therefore requires historicizing himself.[33]

As an historically-oriented "materialist psychiatry" (22/29), then, schizoanalysis will make carefully selective use of all three materialisms of the modern era.[34] The terminology of *Anti-Oedipus*, as we have said, forges connections between Freud's concept of libido and Marx's concept of labor-power; yet it is Nietzsche's concept of will-to-power that cements the relation between them, and enables Deleuze and Guattari to revise psychoanalysis and free repetition from the compulsive form given it by Freud's death instinct. At the same time, Nietzsche and Freud provide a crucial corrective to Marx by supplementing his analysis of exploitation with the analysis of guilt: money is no longer conceived solely as a means of exchange and accumulation, but also as a means of imposing debt and guilt. Consequently, just as there are distinct modes of production for Marx, so are there distinct modes of guilt-formation, linked to what Deleuze and Guattari will call modes of "anti-production"; what psychoanalysis is able to show in this connection is that the nuclear family imposes a modern form of guilt that is neither truly political nor economic in nature. Schizoanalysis therefore concludes that the problems of contemporary social life are not amenable to the kinds of solutions proposed by Nietzsche and Marx taken by themselves: the projects of ending asceticism and nihilism through politico-cultural change and ending exploitation and alienation through socio-economic change both need to take libido and the crushing of desire by the nuclear family into account. Yet if it is the critique of familial guilt that enables schizoanalysis to successfully negotiate a link between Marx's critique of capitalism and Nietzsche's critique of asceticism, it is Marx in turn who enables Deleuze and Guattari to situate historically the characteristically modern forms of familial and cultural guilt in relation to the market and its tendency to substitute the abstract and impersonal calculus of the cash nexus for meaning and authority as the basis of social organization.

It would be a mistake to consider schizoanalysis a grandiose synthesis of these three materialisms (for a synthesis of three such disparate perspectives is probably impossible): they are reciprocally corrective rather than summative or complementary, and may be better understood as forming a pattern of interference with one another rather than a combined conceptual edifice. Yet if the central question to be answered about *Anti-Oedipus* is "how does it work," it must be said that it does not and could not work without drawing selectively on Marx and Freud and Nietzsche (and others), in the ways just outlined. That having been said about the Marx–Nietzsche–Freud nexus in general, we can now return to delineate three key concepts or critical operators that enable *Anti-Oedipus* to perform crucial tasks in developing schizoanalysis as a revolutionary materialist psychiatry.

How it works (2): the critical operators drawn from Kant, Marx, and Freud

Operator 1: Kant and critique

Only after they have completed their presentation of "the connective synthesis of production" on the last page of Chapter Two, Section Three (75/89), do Deleuze and Guattari explain the nature of the "materialist revolution" schizoanalysis performs on psychoanalysis. It is here that the Oedipus is finally identified as precisely the *metaphysics* of psychoanalysis, and where Kant's critique of metaphysics is invoked to illustrate by analogy their own procedure. This is not the place to examine Kantian philosophy in detail; what can be said is this: based on the so-called "Copernican revolution" in epistemology, and speaking in the name of reason, Kant had asserted that the conscious mind utilizes a specific set of processes (which he called the "syntheses of apprehension, reproduction, and recognition") to arrive at knowledge, and had insisted furthermore that whatever did not conform to these processes would stand condemned as metaphysical. Of crucial importance for Kant was the idea that, since these processes were *constitutive* of conscious thought, they provided *immanent* criteria for judging something to be either knowledge or metaphysics, depending on whether it was based on legitimate or illegitimate use of the three syntheses.[35] In a perhaps unfortunate choice of wording, Kant called the illegitimate metaphysical uses of the syntheses "transcendent" (as opposed to "immanent"), and his philosophical critique of metaphysics, "transcendental"; following Kantian usage, then, Deleuze and Guattari call their critique of psychoanalytic metaphysics a "transcendental" critique: it will proceed by distinguishing immanent from metaphysical operations in the unconscious.

In a similar way, but speaking not in the name of reason but in that of desire and especially schizophrenic desire, Deleuze and Guattari insist that the unconscious operates according to a specific set of syntheses to process

14

or constitute experience, and that psychoanalysis must either be shown to conform to these processes or else stand condemned as metaphysical.[36] The early sections of Chapter One present the three syntheses constituting unconscious "thought" (the connective synthesis of production, the disjunctive synthesis of recording, and the conjunctive synthesis of consumption–consummation [*consommation*]), and provide the criteria for distinguishing between their legitimate and illegitimate use. The bulk of Chapter Two then demonstrates, on the basis of these immanent criteria, that Oedipal psychoanalysis is indeed metaphysical, that it makes systematic illegitimate use of the syntheses of the unconscious. Schizoanalysis is thus critical in a Kantian sense, whereas psychoanalysis is not.

Remarkably, this "internal" critique of psychoanalysis not only shows from the "inside" how the Oedipus belies the true nature of the unconscious, but also reveals that the illegitimate Oedipal use of the syntheses is rigorously systematic; Chapter Three will then show from the "outside" that this *system* of Oedipal misrepresentation makes psychoanalysis a strictly capitalist institution. Schizoanalysis thus involves social as well as epistemo-psychological critique: if schizoanalysis condemns psychoanalysis as metaphysical, it will be so condemned as a reflection or projection of capitalism; as an historical-materialist psychiatry, schizoanalysis will call not just for psychoanalytic doctrine but for social relations in general to conform to the syntheses of the unconscious. Schizoanalysis is thus revolutionary in a Marxist sense, whereas psychoanalysis is not. Yet here Deleuze and Guattari's Marxist analyses acquire a distinctly Nietzschean foundation: the social ideal is not what best represents the interests of the proletariat (or humanity as a whole) but what *least* contradicts the "logic" of the unconscious and the active bodily forces animating its syntheses; revolutionary society, too, will have to conform to these unconscious processes or else stand condemned as repressive.

Operator 2: Marx and revolutionary autocritique

If the first frame of reference makes schizoanalysis critical in the Kantian sense of the term, the second frame of reference then makes it critical and revolutionary in a Marxist sense: "schizoanalysis," Deleuze and Guattari insist after presenting and recapitulating the three syntheses of the unconscious, "is at once a transcendental and a materialist analysis" (109/130). The epistemological or (in the Kantian sense) "transcendental" critique just reviewed gets incorporated into an historical-materialist critique which entails "lead[ing] Oedipus to the point of its own autocritique" (109/130). It is only on the last page of Chapter Three, however, that the full scope of this notion of revolutionary autocritique becomes clear: "Freud," they declare, "is the Luther and the Adam Smith of psychiatry" (271/323); so just as Marx brought bourgeois political economy to the point of autocritique, schizoanalysis brings bourgeois psychiatry, i.e. psychoanalysis, to the point of its own autocritique.[37]

This deceptively simple analogy harbors an extraordinary set of claims about history, capitalism, psychoanalysis, and schizoanalysis. For part of what makes schizoanalysis an historical-materialist criticism in the strict Marxist sense is the claim that certain historical conditions made Freud's discovery of the concept of libido possible, just as certain historical conditions made possible Adam Smith and Ricardo's discovery of the concept of labor. And, ultimately, Deleuze and Guattari will claim that the very same conditions were responsible for both. Alone among French poststructuralists in this, they thus not only accept Marx's now controversial position on the relation of capitalism to a "universal history" but actually extend it to include psychoanalysis (understood, again, as a strictly capitalist institution).[38] On their reading, Marx's sense of universal history, because it insists on "its contingent, singular existence, its irony, and its own critique" (271/323), is in effect already a "poststructuralist" one, quite unlike the neo-Hegelian totalizing universal history usually attributed to him (as we shall see in Chapter 4).[39]

In brief, Marx argues that the abstract category of labor-in-general becomes possible in the *thought* of Smith and Ricardo because nascent capitalism has produced abstract labor-in-general in *reality* as soon as workers are separated from means of production and sell their labor-power as a commodity. Abstract labor actually attains real existence under such circumstances, because labor has become an interchangeable commodity on the market; workers themselves have become expendable, the work they do no longer their own: the concrete, objective determination of the workers' labor-power (its transformation from exchange-value into actual use-value) supervenes only *after* it has been purchased as a commodity and is set to work on means of production that remain external to it, as the private property of capitalists. It was at this point historically, Marx reflects, that – like Luther, who defined religion not in terms of institutional objects of worship but as personal and interior religious fervor or faith – Smith and Ricardo define wealth no longer as an objective property of valuable objects but in terms of a subjective essence belonging to productive activity in general – a generality that coincided with capitalism's promotion of abstractly quantified labor-time as the measure of social value. But then, just as Luther re-alienates free subjective religiosity back onto the authority of the Scriptures, so do Smith and Ricardo effectively re-alienate the subjective essence of wealth right back onto private property. And of course so does capitalism itself: labor is subordinated to the "dead hand" of capital as its ultimate determination under capitalism. Hence Smith and Ricardo do not represent critical political economy in the Marxian sense, since they merely *reflect* the apparent objective movement of capitalist society.[40]

So the historical appearance of abstract labor in reality under capitalism constitutes only a *precondition* for a universal history, according to Marx, not its actual foundation; and this in two senses.[41] First of all, capitalism does not constitute a *substantive* foundation for universal history (whereby other modes of production would secretly resemble capitalism), because it is different from, not the same as, all other modes of production: no other social formation "frees" labor from objective pre-determination by making it a commodity; labor appears as a real abstraction only at the end of the process leading up to capitalism.[42] More important, that historical process has not actually reached its end: labor has been freed from objective pre-determination under capitalism only to be *re*-enslaved, at the moment of its sale as a commodity, to external determination by capital.[43] The result is that labor continually reproduces its alienated and alienating conditions of enslavement on an ever-larger scale, as Marx's critique demonstrates. Whereas the apparent objective movement of capital is merely reflected in the representations of Ricardo and Smith, with Marx's critique of bourgeois political economy capitalism attains the point of autocritique and history can become universal: humankind can now envisage and set itself the task of freeing productive activity from any and all external, alien determinations – including the most subtle, abstract, and impersonal of all, that of capital itself.

In relation to this historical pattern of potentially liberating discovery and subsequent re-alienation in Luther and Adam Smith, Deleuze and Guattari insist that "the same thing must be said of Freud" – who is thus understood as "the Luther and the Adam Smith of psychiatry":

> his greatness lies in having determined the essence or nature of desire, no longer in relation to objects, aims or even sources...but as an abstract, subjective essence – libido or sexuality. But he still relates this essence to the family [and to]...Oedipus.
>
> (270/322)

Even after discovering the nature of passion not in relation to its objects or aims but rather as indeterminate desire, as libidinal energy in general, Freud then betrays the logic of the unconscious by re-alienating desire onto the Oedipus complex and subordinating it to the family triangle as its ultimate determination. Psychoanalysis, too, thus merely reflects the apparent objective movement of the nuclear family, itself a product of capitalism, and does not attain the point of autocritique.

So just as capitalism makes universal history possible through its difference rather than its identity – by freeing productive activity in principle from all previous forms of external pre-determination, even though it in fact re-subjects labor to capital as the most abstract form of external determination – so do the Oedipus and Oedipal psychoanalyses similarly participate in universal history: not – *pace* Freud – as themselves the universal form and truth of desire, but through the recognition in principle of untrammeled desire as abstract subjective essence, as libido, despite the subsequent re-enslavement of that desire in fact and in theory to the nuclear family and the Oedipus as its most private and abstract metaphysical representation. "Yes," Deleuze and Guattari allow, despite the title of their book, "Oedipus is nevertheless the universal of desire, the product of universal history – but on one condition, which is not met by Freud: that Oedipus be capable...of conducting its autocritique" (271/323).[44] In schizoanalysis, the Oedipus becomes capable at last of conducting its autocritique.

Operator 3: Freud and the tendentious joke

This is not to say, however, that Marx and Freud made the same discovery: desire and labor are evidently *not* the "same thing"; indeed, maintaining their specific difference is, as we have seen, one of the key traits distinguishing schizoanalysis from others' attempts to connect Marx and Freud. Yet Deleuze and Guattari do claim that both discoveries were made possible by specific historical conditions, namely the emergence of capitalism: as they put it, "the discovery of production *in general and without distinction*, as it appears in capitalism, is the identical discovery of *both* political economy *and* psychoanalysis, beyond the determinate systems of representation" (302/360). Schizoanalysis, in other words, will want to translate desire and labor from their respective "determinate systems of representation" (psycho-analysis and political economy) into the concepts of "desiring-production" and "social-production," precisely in order to stress their common deriva-tion from "production in general and without distinction" as it appears under capitalism.

Yet the emergence of capitalism not only made the discovery of desire and labor possible but also produced the *segregation of domains* in which each came to exist as a distinct entity with a corresponding determinate system of representation: the realm of "production" – specifically of commodity-production – on one hand, and the realm of "reproduction" – including biological but also psychological reproduction – on the other. Production-in-general in both domains, in other words, is subject under capitalism to a radical and alienating *privatization*: to capital as agent of privatized production; to the nuclear family as organization of privatized reproduction. So one of the main tasks of *Anti-Oedipus*, we learn in the last chapter, will be to demonstrate

> why, at the same time [that] it discovers the subjective essence of
> desire and labor – a common essence inasmuch as it is the activity
> of production in general...capitalism [is] continually re-alienating
> this essence...in a repressive machine that divides the essence in two,
> and maintains it divided – abstract labor on one hand, abstract

desire on the other: political economy and psychoanalysis, political economy and libidinal economy.

(302–3/360)

The identity-and-difference of production-in-general constitutes the third critical frame of reference organizing *Anti-Oedipus*. Deleuze and Guattari insist that there is an "identity of nature" between social-production and desiring-production, but also a "difference in regime."[45] The difference in regime enables schizoanalysis to critique the organization of social-production in the name of desiring-production (as will become clear in Chapter 2), once their identity of nature is realized. And ironically enough (as we will see in Chapter 4), their identity of nature becomes visible only under capitalism where the difference in regime between the two is most pronounced.

Indeed, the book's very chapter divisions – which separate the critique of the "holy family" (Chapter Two) from the typology of modes of social organization (Chapter Three) – emphasize the difference in regime, reproducing rather than reconciling the capitalist segregation of desire from labor. So the link between desire and labor will in the first place be forged *lexically*, instead: such is the function of the concept of desiring-machines itself, along with other schizoanalytic terms like "deterritorialization" and "reterritorialization," "decoding" and "recoding," and "desiring-production." And it is through this lexical counterpoint to the chapter divisions that the book functions overall as a tendentious joke, as we shall see. But first it is important to show how the concepts created by Deleuze and Guattari serve to link the domains of social- and desiring-production, and thus reveal their identical nature despite the difference in regime.

"Territorialization" is a term derived from Lacan's analysis of the process by which parental care-giving, starting with maternal breast-feeding, maps the infant's erogenous zones, charging specific organs and corresponding objects with erotic energy and value (the lips and the breast, for example). Territorialization thus programs desire to valorize certain organs and objects at the expense of others, and at the expense of what Freud called "polymorphous perversity": the free-flowing, relatively unfixed, form of desire Deleuze and Guattari call schizophrenia. As one would expect, the schizoanalytic term "*de*territorialization" designates, in the psychological register, the reverse of Lacanian territorialization – that is to say, the process of freeing desire from established organs and objects: one of the principal aims of schizoanalysis, for example, is to free schizophrenic desire from the nuclear family and from the oedipal representations of desire promulgated by psychoanalysis. At the same time, however, Deleuze and Guattari use "deterritorialization" – now in the social register – to designate the freeing of labor-power from specific means of production, as in the case of English peasants who were banished or "freed" by the Enclosure Acts (1709–1869) from common land when it was enclosed for sheep-grazing. Some peasants, of course, would eventually find jobs working at looms in the nascent textile industry: their labor-power was thereby re-attached or "reterritorialized" onto new means of production. The processes of deterritorialization and reterritorialization accompany the fundamental mechanism of capital, "axiomatization": it operates by conjoining deterritorialized resources and appropriating the surplus arising from their reterritorializing conjunction. The original capitalist axiom, for example, conjoined deterritorialized wealth – i.e. monetary wealth no longer embodied in landed property – with deterritorialized labor-power bereft of any means of subsistence: the axiomatization of these deterritorialized flows linked liquid wealth invested in means of production with "free" workers with nothing to sell but their labor-power. Subsequently, the continuing development of capitalism has axiomatized many other resource-flows – including knowledge, skills, and taste – and integrated them into the production process.

Indeed, incessant cycles of deterritorialization and reterritorialization through axiomatization constitute one of the fundamental rhythms of capitalist society as a whole – what Marx referred to as the "constant revolutionizing of the means of production [and] uninterrupted disturbance of all social conditions [that] distinguish the bourgeois epoch from all earlier ones"[46]: capital is extracted from one locale (the rust belt, the United States) and re-invested somewhere else (the south, the Pacific rim); labor skills corresponding to certain means of production are, for a time, fostered and well paid, only to become worthless a few years later when new means of production prevail; consumer preferences are first programmed by advertising to value one set of goods, only to be deprogrammed so as to consider them "out of fashion," and reprogrammed by another advertising campaign to value a "new" set of goods. The terms deterritorialization and reterritorialization thus presuppose and reinforce the notice of a "common essence...of desire and labor," referring without distinction to the detachment and reattachment of the energies of "production in general" (including "consumption") to objects of investment of all kinds, whether conventionally considered "psychological" or "economic."

Closely linked with deterritorialization and reterritorialization are the parallel terms "decoding" and "recoding," which bear on representations rather than on concrete objects. Decoding, it is important to note, does not refer to the process of translating a secret meaning or message into clearer form: on the contrary, it refers to a process of dis-investing given meanings altogether, to a process of "uncoding," if you like: the destabilization and ultimately the elimination of established codes that confer fixed meaning. If capitalism deterritorializes because of the imperative to constantly revolutionize production and consumption so as to generate and realize surplus-value, it decodes because it defines and measures value in terms of abstract quantities, because its basic institution is the market. It thus bears comparison with Weber's and especially Lukács's notions of rationalization and reification, as already suggested. Chapter Three of *Anti-Oedipus* shows that whereas other societies are based on codes, on the establishment of qualitative similarities that underlie stable meanings, capitalism systematically undermines codes, replacing them with the cash nexus of the market as the basis of social organization. Alone among French poststructuralists, Deleuze and Guattari thus provide an historical, materialist ground for the by-now-familiar tenet of the instability of meaning as well as for the preference for difference over identity: both are effects of the decoding process characteristic of capitalism.[47]

The symmetry implied in the corresponding term "recoding," however, is somewhat misleading; the term in fact rarely appears in *Anti-Oedipus*.[48] This is because capitalist axiomatization, according to Deleuze and Guattari, is ultimately a *meaningless* calculus involving purely abstract quantities: "the capitalist machine is incapable of providing a code that will apply to the whole of the social field" (33/41). Were it not for the inconvenience of having human workers, managers, and consumers, capitalism might do very nicely without any meanings whatsoever. The belief in any *general* meaning under these conditions is hopelessly nostalgic and obsolete – or "paranoid," in the specific sense Deleuze and Guattari intend. Whatever temporary local meanings capitalism does provide through recoding are strictly derivative of the axioms that happen to be in place: job-training and re-training programs, for instance, provide certain local meanings associated with manual labor; research projects in academic or corporate labs provide other meanings for intellectual work; taste-management through advertising provides still others for consumption, and so on. But they never "add up" to a stable global code or system of meanings: under capitalism, decoding prevails. That is why schizoanalysis takes schizophrenia – creative semiosis unlimited by fixed meaning – to be the fundamental tendency under capitalism and the promise of freedom in universal history, while the tendency to paranoia appears as a reaction-formation derived from the forced privatization of "productive activity in general," in economics and family-life alike.

Given this imbalance between decoding and recoding and the relative insignificance of meaning under capitalism, it is no wonder that deterritorialization, axiomatization, and reterritorialization are more fundamental analytic categories for schizoanalysis, since they bear on material objects and processes rather than meanings.[49] Yet for the purposes of comparing decoded capitalist society with other societies (in Chapter 3) and situating Lacan's structural–linguistic version of psychoanalysis in historical context, the categories of decoding and recoding are crucial to the schizoanalytic endeavor: they provide a materialist semiotics, as it were, to accompany its materialist psychiatry and political economy.

The concept of "desiring-machines," finally, while serving cognitively to connect libido and labor in a single term as we have said, also serves key polemical purposes. Foremost among these will be to replace the theater

model of the psyche found throughout Freud with a factory model. This constitutes for one thing a rejection of tragedy (as in *Oedipus Rex*, *Hamlet*, and so
on) as an appropriate mode for the analytic endeavor: schizoanalytic therapy,
were such a thing to exist, would end with a hearty chuckle, not a rueful sigh.
In any case, schizoanalysis effects a Nietzschean transvaluation of psychoanalysis by eliminating its pervasive sense of guilt and tragic resignation to
defeat and death, in favor of affirmation of the forces of life. More important, Deleuze and Guattari reject representation itself – in theatrical or any
other form – as a distortion of the real mode of operation of the unconscious,
which is productive rather than expressive or representative: "The unconscious poses no problems of meaning, solely problems of use. The question
posed by desire is not 'What does it mean?' but '*How does it work?*'"(109/129)

In fact, Deleuze and Guattari consider representation to be not just a
distortion of desire but *the principal means of repressing desire* and of
betraying its authentic schizophrenic form. Even if the answer given by
psychoanalysis did not endlessly revolve around the "Oedipus complex," the
very question of "what desire means" already entails a profound misunderstanding of the unconscious: whenever and however it is answered, it traps
desire in repressive representations of one kind or another. The factory
model of desire thus forms part of Deleuze and Guattari's contribution to
the "critique of representation" that constitutes such an important part of
French poststructuralism.

The other major polemical target of the factory model of productive
desire is the widespread view – stretching from Plato all the way up to and
including Freud and Lacan – which defines desire in terms of *lack*. Here
again, Deleuze and Guattari draw inspiration from Nietzschean affirmation:
desire, they insist, does not lack anything, does not aim at what it does not
have or what is "missing"; it does not construct a fantasy-world containing
objects of desire apart and different from the real world. On the contrary,
desire is first and foremost productive force, and what it produces is simply
the real world: "If desire produces, its product is real. If desire is productive,
it can be productive only in the real world and can produce only reality....
The objective being of desire is the Real in and of itself" (26–7/34).[50] Only
secondarily, as a result of social organizations which deprive certain people
or classes of their objective being and the fruits of their labor, does productive desire become reactive and construct a parallel world of gratification
(sometimes called "fantasy," sometimes "heaven") as *imaginary compensa-
tion* for what has been taken from it.[51] To the extent that psychoanalysis
subscribes to the notion that desire is based on lack rather than on force,
Deleuze and Guattari consider it a reactive, *slave* psychology; under the
cloak of the psychoanalyst, as Nietzsche might say, they smell a *priest*.[52]

To claim that *labor* "produces" reality is one thing – and fairly common-
place: Hegel, Vico, and Marx all supply versions of such a claim. But to claim
that *desire* produces reality is something else. It resembles, in one respect,

claims made in phenomenology – but without the "epoché," the famous brack-eting of claims to objective reality: phenomenologists study the "things them-selves" as they are constituted by human attention or intention, without regard for their correspondence (or lack of correspondence) with "objective reality" as defined by science. For schizoanalysis, of course, it is unconscious rather than conscious "intention" that constitutes reality. But more import-ant, the difference between the "phenomenologically constituted" real and the "scientific" real is strictly secondary, according to schizoanalysis: both "versions" of reality are first of all products of desire, before distinctions between them can be drawn (distinctions which, as Nietzsche would insist, are themselves also products of a certain kind of desire!).

A better sense of the active force of productive desire may be gleaned from forensic usage; desire produces reality in the same sense that lawyers "produce" evidence in a court of law: they cannot "wish" it into existence; they don't make it up, but they do make it count as real. Here, too, however, any distinction between what counts as fact, evidence, and reality inside the courtroom and what counts outside it is moot: desire in the schizoanalytic sense produces reality in and of itself, *before* any such inside–outside distinc-tions can be drawn. Given this Nietzschean transvaluation of desire as active force, the connection forged by the concept of desiring-machines between desire and labor should appear less perplexing. Through the investment of energy in psychic as well as physical form, desiring-machines produce reality, both in the cognitive sense of psychic drives shaping the phenomenal world and in the economic sense of labor-power shaping the material world.

The notion of the productivity of desire implied by the term desiring-machines thus reconnects what capitalism divides in two, namely "the sub-jective essence of desire and labor...inasmuch as it is the activity of prod-uction in general" (302/360). Yet precisely because capitalism objectively divides in two the subjective essence of production, *Anti-Oedipus* as a critique of capitalism must analyze the difference between the two at the same time that it exposes it as factitious. Schizoanalysis therefore insists that while desire and labor are essentially the same productive force, they nonetheless operate under capitalism according to different regimes, which are conventionally mapped by different disciplines: political economy and psychoanalysis. Although Deleuze and Guattari show little respect for the boundary sepa-rating these two disciplines, they do maintain a specific difference between the regimes themselves, which they refer to as desiring-production (formerly libido) and social-production (labor). But this difference is not between fantasy and reality: "There is no such thing as the social production of reality on the one hand, and a desiring-production that is mere fantasy on the other...*social production is purely and simply desiring-production itself under determinate conditions*" (28–9/36). In this light, we can better understand the basic thrust and organization of *Anti-Oedipus*.

For by insisting lexically on the identical nature of social- and desiring-production beneath their difference in regime under capitalism, Deleuze and Guattari in effect set up their *Anti-Oedipus* as one big joke: more precisely, as what Freud calls a tendentious joke. As he explains in *Jokes and their Relation to the Unconscious*, jokes of this kind work by surreptitiously linking two topics or domains that logical, "mature" thought normally keeps separate through repression. In making a sudden and unexpected link between them, often by means of a lexical shortcut such as a play on words or *double-entendre*, the tendentious joke produces pleasure by obviating the effort of repression keeping them separate (Freud says that we laugh off the quota of now-useless repressive energy), while simultaneously smuggling the attack on its intended target past the censor. Such is precisely the effect of the lexical link Deleuze and Guattari forge between desiring-production and social-production through their use of the term *desiring-machines*: the normally distinct regimes of libidinal economy and political economy, of asceticism and capitalism, are targeted by a mode of critique that simultaneously produces pleasure and insight by showing that these economies are in fact one and the same. This helps explain the glee and exhilaration with which Deleuze and Guattari mount their attack on psychoanalysis, capitalism, and the Oedipus.

More practically speaking, the relation between desiring-production and social-production illuminates the divisions of the book itself. Chapter Three examines three types of determinate historical conditions under which social-production and therefore desiring-production are shown to operate in significantly different ways. It constitutes an "external" critique of the Oedipus by performing a genealogy to show where, socio-historically, the Oedipus came from, what forms it took in previous societies, and how it gets transformed and realized under capitalism through the privatization of reproduction in the nuclear family. Chapter Two constitutes an "internal" critique of the Oedipus, showing how it betrays the schizophrenia of the desiring-machines presented in Chapter One by trapping it in Oedipal representations arising objectively from the institution of the nuclear family, as well as from psychoanalysis itself. Chapter Four then sets out a program for schizoanalysis based on its critique of psychoanalysis in Chapter Two and its transformation of historical materialism in Chapter Three. For clarity of presentation, this study will retain the distinction between the "internal" and "external" critiques of the Oedipus, devoting a chapter to each one, but will return to the critique of the family and psychoanalysis as specifically capitalist institutions at the end of Chapter Three, with a better understanding of the determinate conditions under which the Oedipus arrived historically under capitalism and then reached the point of autocritique in schizoanalysis.

2

DESIRING-PRODUCTION AND
THE INTERNAL CRITIQUE OF
OEDIPUS

The schizoanalytic model of the psyche is that of a machine, or a set of machines: the desiring-machines. Describing it is one of the most important tasks of this book, since both the internal and the external critiques of the Oedipus follow directly from the ways schizoanalysis understands the psyche to operate. It is also one of the most difficult tasks, and I ask readers to bear with me for the next few pages. In the hope of facilitating comprehension, I have separated the presentation of the model from its mobilization in the critique of Oedipus. The disadvantage of such a gambit is that the model standing alone will appear somewhat abstract; the advantage is that we will be able to concentrate on the model itself before it is brought to bear on aspects of psychoanalysis that are often complex and difficult to understand in their own right.

The desiring-machines operate according to three syntheses, called the connective synthesis of production, the disjunctive synthesis of recording (*enregistrement*), and the conjunctive synthesis of consumption–consummation (*consommation*).[1] Deleuze and Guattari refer to these modes of psychic functioning as "syntheses," in part to invoke the analogy with Kant's "syntheses of apperception," as was said in Chapter 1; but the term also draws on Deleuze's effort in *Difference and Repetition* to build on Freud's recognition of the importance of repetition in psychic life by recasting it in terms of a materialist ontology of repetition where difference instead of similarity prevails, as we shall see in a moment. As a first approximation, we can say that the syntheses are ways of processing or indeed constituting experience (in much the same way that Kant's syntheses of apperception are ways of constituting knowledge). The connective synthesis concerns instincts and drives, and the ways they endow objects with value or erotic charge; roughly speaking, it translates Freud's notion of libidinal investment or *cathexis* and the functions he assigns to Eros or the life instinct. The disjunctive synthesis involves the functioning of pleasure, memory, and signs in the psyche, along with what Freud called the death instinct, or Thanatos. The conjunctive synthesis, finally, is about the formation of subjectivity. We now need to examine in more detail how these syntheses work and how they fit together. We will then be in a position to understand what purposes such a description of the psyche serves in the schizoanalytic endeavor.

The three syntheses of the unconscious

The connective synthesis of production

The connective synthesis of production is in some ways the easiest of the three to understand, deriving as it does from the Freudian notions of "drive," psychic "investment" (*investissement*) or "cathexis," and "polymorphous perversity." Productive desire makes connections, and what it connects are part-objects (often but not necessarily organs). An infant's mouth at the breast constitutes such a connection, but so do the relations between an eye and a breast, an eye and a face, an eye and a knee; and between a mouth and a bottle, a mouth and an iron-lung, a mouth and the atmosphere, a mouth and a finger, a finger and a lock of hair (even though some of these latter do not involve organs alone). For now, three features are essential. In the first place, the production of such connections corresponds to Freudian drives and constitutes the materialist basis of the model: connections are made so as to tap into a source of energy and procure a "charge," whether physiological, erotic, or both. Second, syntheses of production connect only what Melanie Klein termed "part-objects," not whole persons or organs understood as belonging to whole persons.[2] If an infant's mouth connects to a mother's breast while at the same time its eye scans her face, the synthesis of production makes only those two connections: the breast and face are not connected to one another nor to a larger whole, are not viewed as belonging to a single whole person. Third, the connections made by the synthesis of production are multiple, heterogeneous, and continual: an eye scans a head of hair, and then sees a face, and then a breast, and then a knee; a mouth connects to a breast, to some air, and then to a finger; a finger connects to a lock of hair, and then to a mouth, and so on. Deleuze and Guattari thus sum up the syntax of the connective synthesis as a series of "and...and then...and then..." (5/11) whereby one "organ–machine" (6/12) connects with another, and then another, and then another[3] – provided we understand the semantics of the term "organ" being used here to qualify these machines in the broadest possible "polymorphous" way, as any partial-object which gives or gets a charge or flow of energy through a connection.

The disjunctive synthesis of recording

The disjunctive synthesis of recording is more complicated. The notion that the psyche contains a recording-apparatus is nothing new: Freud himself, for example, found it useful to construct a model of the psyche based on the analogy with a "mystic writing pad"; on a more general level, he suggested that drives invest (or cathect) mentally recorded images of previous objects of satisfaction whenever the organism cannot obtain the objects themselves.[4] Deleuze and Guattari attach even more importance to processes of recording in the psyche, and will thereby bring the poststructuralist critique of representation to bear on psychoanalysis and its fixation on the Oedipus complex. To account for recording processes in the psyche, Deleuze and Guattari will develop the concept of the "body-without-organs" (a term derived from Antonin Artaud[5]) and dramatically transform the notion of the "death instinct" that Freud had developed in one of his most radically speculative works, *Beyond the Pleasure Principle*. As crucial as these concepts are to schizoanalysis, they are among the most difficult to understand, in large part because the re-writing of the death instinct and at least an adumbration of the body-without-organs are accomplished in *Difference and Repetition*, written before Deleuze began collaborating with Guattari, and are to some extent taken for granted in *Anti-Oedipus*. This is not the place to examine in detail the argument of *Difference and Repetition*, a work of extraordinary complexity in its own right, but it is important nonetheless to review its contributions to the strategic arsenal of *Anti-Oedipus*.

The aim of *Difference and Repetition*, Deleuze's major contribution to a materialist philosophy of poststructuralism, is to restore the concept of "difference" to its rightful place in relation to "identity."[6] Extending lines of argument from Nietzsche, and using them against most of the Western metaphysical tradition from Plato onwards, Deleuze insists that difference and multiplicity are the primary categories, and that identity is secondary and dependent on them, rather than the other way around. Difference and multiplicity are what is given ontologically; they then get betrayed and distorted by operations (including, notably, the Hegelian "work of the negative") that result in identity. Restoring the category of difference to its rightful place of primacy in turn transforms the concept of "repetition," for it is henceforth necessary to understand repetition to involve not identity or equivalence among terms, but difference and variation. Within a materialist ontology of difference, what gets repeated is not the same, but different.

Freud is of great interest in this connection: he insisted that repetition was central to the psyche, but nevertheless conceived of repetition in metaphysical rather than materialist terms – as repetition of the same. According to the Freud of *Beyond the Pleasure Principle*, the compulsion to repeat is what makes pleasure a principle of psychic life: we take pleasure in what we have previously found to be pleasurable. Yet since Freud's repetition compulsion is grounded in a death instinct that stipulates a "return to the inorganic state" of matter before life began, it is ultimately governed by identity, by a mechanical return to the same, rather than by difference. Freud's instincts are therefore, as he himself put it, "innately conservative"; even the pleasure principle, on this understanding of repetition, succumbs to stasis, fixation, neurosis. Restoring difference to repetition does not diminish the importance of repetition in psychic life as the principle of pleasure, but frees pleasure from mechanical repetition and a strictly linear temporality: whereas repetition of the same constitutes a static neurotic form of pleasure fixed on the past, the repetition of difference takes pleasure in variation, ramification, improvisation (as these are achieved by the exercise of active force).[7]

We can now return to the schizoanalytic syntheses of desire, for taking pleasure in variation and ramification rather than in mechanical repetition requires a complementary counter-force to the connective synthesis, which would otherwise lock the organism into instinctual or habitual patterns of connection. Such a counter-force would allow a given set of organ–machine connections to be broken and other connections made in their place, only to be broken in their turn and replaced with others, and so on *ad infinitum*.

> Desiring-machines [operating by connective synthesis] make us an organism; but at the very heart of production, within the very production of this production [of organ-machine connections], the body suffers from being organized in this way, from not having some other organization, or no organization at all....The [machines] stop dead and set free the unorganized mass [of energy-flows] they once served to articulate.
>
> (8/14)

This is the role of Deleuze and Guattari's version of the death instinct: to bring productive desire to a halt, to suspend or freeze the connections it has made, in order that new and different connections may become possible; they therefore prefer the term "anti-production" to "death instinct" (and will go on to show in Chapter Three how anti-production under capitalism comes to appear as an "instinct" and gets misunderstood as such by psychoanalysis).[8] The effect of anti-production on the connective syntheses, then, is to desexualize desire by neutralizing the organ-machine connections, and thereby constitute a surface that records networks of relations among connections, instead of producing connections themselves: it is this recording-surface that Deleuze and Guattari refer to as the body-without-organs.[9]

It should now be clearer why they resort to this obscure term borrowed from Artaud: it is used to raise the question of how the body is organ-ized, and how it might be actively dis-organ-ized so as to enable the production of other forms of organ-ization – or no fixed organ-ization at all, which is the state they designate as schizophrenia. Schizoanalysis construes the body as an assemblage of "organs" in the broadest sense of the term, including not just sex and sense organs, but all parts of the body that either focalize sensations and feelings of pleasure or pain, or perform actions of use or expenditure: the tongue as organ of taste but also as organ of speech and song; the opposable thumb as organ for grasping an ax but also for operating a track-ball or signaling someone's death. Yet along with its organ-ization of organs, the body as schizoanalysis construes it also has a force and a locus of dis-organ-ization – anti-production and the body-without-organs – which can prevent any given organ-ization from becoming permanently fixed.[10] Whether fixed organ-ization or radical dis-organ-ization is likely to prevail depends ultimately on the mode of social-production and one's place in or stance toward it, as will become clear in Chapter 3.

The formation of the body-without-organs opens or subjects animal instinct to the distinctively human form of time: to memory and to repetition. What registers on the body-without-organs are essentially signs of organ-machine connections that enable or oblige us to repeat previous modes of desiring-satisfaction, albeit with greater or lesser degrees of freedom of variation within repetition. Forming a system of relations, these signs bind or synthesize time, enabling us to relate or compare one satisfaction to another, and to take pleasure not necessarily in experiencing the new in terms of the old (as Freud would have it) but simply in experiencing one thing in relation to something else, instead. For inasmuch as the signs comprise a "system of possible permutations among differences" (12/18; translation modified) on the body-without-organs, they bind time synchronically, as Lacan (following Saussure) might put it, rather than linearly.[11]

In fact, Deleuze and Guattari credit Lacan with "the discovery of this fertile domain of a code of the unconscious" (38/46), i.e. an unconscious comprised of signs forming a synchronic differential system. But they insist on several qualifications to this discovery. For one thing, the system of rela-tions formed on the body-without-organs is not linear, does not sponsor what Lacan calls the "metonymy of desire," a vain search for some lost object from the past;[12] it operates instead by a radically indeterminate mode of "free association" among signs. They thus do not, for another, form a single "signifying chain," as Lacan would have it, but many: sign-relations on the body-without-organs form "a multiplicity so complex that we can scarcely speak of one chain or even of one code of desire" (38/46). Finally, not only are these signs not meaningful (as Lacan would ultimately agree), they do not even belong to one sign-system (as Lacan claims they do: the unconscious as language-system); instead they are radically heterogeneous, and thus

> may include a succession of characters from different alphabets in which an ideogram, a pictogram, a tiny image of an elephant passing by, or a rising sun may suddenly make an appearance. In...mix[ing] together phonemes, morphemes, etc. without combining them, papa's mustache, mama's upraised arm, a ribbon, a little girl, a cop, a shoe suddenly turn up.
>
> (39/47; translation modified)

Synchronic rather than linear or metonymic, multiple rather than singular, heterogeneous and polyvocal rather than univocal and meaningful, "the one vocation of the sign is to produce desire, engineering it in every direction" (39/47). From the multiplicity of sign-relations and the plurality of codes on the body-without-organs, several crucial questions will emerge for the materialist semiotics constituted by schizoanalysis: what directions does desire engineered this way in fact take? Which of the many codes organizing desire tend to prevail? Why do any specific codes have to prevail over others at all?[13] But before or beneath the constitution of such a sign-system, the concept of the body-without-organs raises other questions as well, notably about the nature of its relations to the organ-machine connections that precede and, as it were, fuel it.

Although the term itself is borrowed from Artaud, the concept of the body-without-organs also bears a certain resemblance to Lacan's notion of the "unary trait" which introduces signification into the psyche and thereby creates the Lacanian unconscious.[14] Lacan is interested in the moment at which the human infant leaves the domain of mute, but substantial, material existence and enters the universe of signification. In a suggestive re-reading of Freud's discussion of Little Hans' game of "*fort-da,*" Lacan proposes that the game is not about Little Hans managing his mother's absence, but about his entry into language as a purely differential system lacking any substance whatsoever. Taken in isolation, a sound such as "fort" may entertain a direct relation with an emotional state (e.g. separation-anxiety), as does a cry of pain, but it does not yet signify in a fully meaningful way. Only when it gets paired and contrasted with a different syllable – such as "da" in Little Hans' game – does the sound "fort" become a true signifier, and thereby propel us into the differential universe of signification.

What is crucial for Lacan is that "fort" henceforth plays a role in two registers: in consciousness and the universe of signification, it will eventually take on meaning differentially within a vast network of other signifiers, as merely one substitutable sign among many; in the unconscious, however, it functions as the "unary trait" representing the substantiality of matter "before" the advent of signification, as well as the substantiality of the body "beneath" consciousness. It is thus the founding element of the unconscious. Repression, in Lacan's view, is based on this incompatibility between the substantial nature of the body and bodily drives, on the one hand, and the differential nature of language as signifying system and of consciousness, on the other: being and meaning do not interface or converge; human language fails to represent the human body.

The unary trait henceforth serves as a kind of magnet of lost substantiality, drawing all subsequently repressed material into the unconscious where it forms its own matrix of differential relations: the unconscious is now structured like a language, with a constantly shifting, idiosyncratic set of "meanings" all its own. But for the existentialist psychoanalyst, such meanings are radically groundless and ultimately illusory: as a kind of screen separating differential meaning from bodily substance, the meaningless unary trait blocks access to the body and its drives, which are thus forever tragically "lost" to consciousness. For Deleuze and Guattari, the body-without-organs functions, like the unary trait, as such a screen between the body and consciousness, but with several differences. For one thing, the sign-system constituted on the body-without-organs is not exclusively linguistic, and therefore not purely differential in the sense that Saussure insisted phonetic language is. Moreover, given Deleuze's understanding of the repetition compulsion within his materialist ontology, bodily drives are themselves already differential as well as substantial (and, given Deleuze and Guattari's materialist semiotics, we might add, systems of representation are equally substantial as well as differential). So there is for schizoanalysis no absolute, tragic incompatibility between the body and processes of signification. Instead, the relative compatibility or incompatibility of desire with any historically given system of representation depends on the degree to which that system contravenes or agrees with the modes of operation intrinsic to desire (i.e. operates according to illegitimate or legitimate use of the syntheses). For now what is important is that the body-without-organs represents for schizoanalysis not just the locus of repression but the potential for freedom. It can be compared to a kind of *tabula rasa*, freeing the organism from the purely mechanical repetition of instinctual determination as well as the fixations of neurosis – provided we understand that such a *tabula rasa* does not exist from the start, but rather gets produced in the course of psychic development by the transformation of energies of connection into energies of recording.

The body-without-organs is constituted as a recording-surface in the first place, as I said, when the energy of anti-production de-sexualizes or neutralizes the active connections made by productive desire. In fact, the interplay of desiring-production and anti-production generates alternating rhythms of attraction and repulsion between the organ–machines and the body-without-organs. When anti-production predominates, "the body without organs presents its smooth, slippery, opaque, taut surface as a barrier...in order to resist organ–machines" (9/15). When productive desire prevails, machines "attach themselves to the body-without-organs as so many points of disjunction, between which an entire network of new syntheses is now woven, marking the surface off into co-ordinates, like a grid" (12/18). What is essential is that even while anti-production interrupts or suspends existing productive connections on the body-without-organs, it at the same time registers their diverse possibilities, and ends up multiplying the relations among them to infinity. Hence the importance of the syntax of the disjunctive synthesis of recording, which selects and networks signs of organ–machines produced by connective syntheses in a strictly open-ended series: "either...or...or...."

Unlike Freud, for whom a recording-apparatus emerges in the psyche because infantile desire hampered by lack of motor control is unable to obtain the real object of gratification and therefore invests ("hallucinatory") images of satisfaction instead; and unlike Lacan, for whom the recording-function of the unconscious is based on the unary trait which radically separates bodily drives from consciousness, Deleuze and Guattari see disjunctive synthesis on the body-without-organs first emerging as a trans-formation of connective energy itself, at the point when an identity between the process of desiring-production and a finished product has been achieved.[15] The connection between mouth and breast, for example, gets broken when it has finished producing its "product," which is nourishment or satisfaction: as the connection gives way to disjunction, it registers on the body-without-organs as a sign of satisfaction, and the infant rejects the breast and turns away. The mouth is now freed from the breast, and may lapse into quiescence or become some other organ altogether: an organ for expelling instead of ingesting liquid, for example, if the infant proceeds to burp or vomit; or an organ for smiling; or an organ for expelling a flow of air instead of liquid, if the child sighs happily, or starts to cry or coo or babble.

More significantly, the infant may pull away from the breast for other reasons, without any ultimate physiological satisfaction having been achieved. Perhaps a smile catches its eye, and it suspends the mouth–breast connection to pursue an eye–face connection instead – and then maybe looks away and brings a finger into connection with a lock of hair: in each case the disjunctive energy of anti-production functions to suspend one organ-machine connection, but only for the sake of another, in an open-ended series: either mouth–breast, or eye–smile, or finger–hair, or whatever. The body-without-organs is thus ultimately what frees the human animal from instinctual determination, for it prevents us from remaining fixated on any (developmentally or historically) given mode of satisfaction. What possibilities would exist for the development of culinary arts, for instance, if humans remained exclusively fixated on the breast for nourishment, or for oral gratification? The senses and organs can operate productively (in the broadest sense: creatively; as "theoreticians in their immediate praxis," as Marx put it[16]) only on condition that they are freed from pre-established or instinctual connections and modes of satisfaction – and that is one effect of anti-production: to produce the body-without-organs as a kind of *tabula rasa* on which objects of drives and instincts register so as to multiply and differentiate.

The disjunctive energy of anti-production is not without its dangers, however. Just as the connective energy of desiring-production can succumb to fixation, the disjunctive or repulsive energy of anti-production can lead to total breakdown. If productive connections are systematically broken or denied by others, such denial can subsequently be "internalized" via repression, taken up and reproduced autonomously by the force of anti-production operating consistently against the organism's own connective syntheses: the temporary deferral of gratification associated with self-mastery and the enhancement of active force can become the absolute refusal of gratification characteristic of neurosis and self-denial. Anti-production in the psyche thus corresponds to what Freud called "primal repression," an autonomous counter-force that paves the way for repression properly so-called, which involves interpersonal and social relations.[17] Taken to the extreme, anti-production can prevent the formation of any organ-machine connections whatsoever, thereby bringing about complete withdrawal onto what Deleuze and Guattari sometimes call the "full" body-without-organs: this is the condition known in psychiatry as catatonia – a condition which Deleuze and Guattari suggest is usually the result of capitalist society's violent refusal to countenance the process of schizophrenia fostered by capitalism itself.[18]

The conjunctive synthesis of consumption–consummation

Between the extremes of instinctual determination via mechanical repetition of organ-connections, on the one hand, and catatonic breakdown via complete refusal of organ–machines and withdrawal onto the full body-without-organs, on the other, the interplay of the forces of production and anti-production generate a wide range of familiar personality-types or forms of subjectivity. When production and anti-production conflict systematically, two specific forms of subjectivity result which are noteworthy, in part because Freud had already identified them as corollaries of one another: the neurotic and the pervert.[19] In the neurotic, the forces of anti-production prevail: desiring-production is denied one or more of its own connections and is constrained to fix instead on a relatively ungratifying substitute connection (the neurotic symptom). In the pervert, the forces of production prevail: an unorthodox organ-connection is maintained despite (or, in some cases, because of) social sanctions against it.

Beyond their symmetrical relation with one another, however, the subjects of neurosis and perversion are noteworthy because they illustrate in dramatic or exaggerated form the relation of the third synthesis, the conjunctive synthesis of consumption–consummation, to the interplay of production and anti-production comprising the first two: the subject emerges *only as an after-effect* of the selections made by desire among various disjunctive and connective syntheses, *not as the agent* of selection. Neurotics and perverts are not so by conscious choice; they are not the agents but the results of connections and disjunctions made on the body-without-organs by the interplay of forces of production and anti-production that constitute them as subjects. Similarly, when the infant rejects the breast and turns away to smile at a familiar face, this act is not chosen by but constitutes the infant as a subject (as "a snacker," "an extrovert," or whatever).

"Normal" adults, by contrast, typically indulge in the illusion – the metaphysics of sovereign subjectivity – whereby they choose their pleasures and desires, rather than being "chosen," that is to say constituted, by them; Deleuze and Guattari draw directly on Nietzsche to dispel this illusion and insist that the productions and anti-productions of desire, like "will-to-power," always come first, and the appearance of the subject afterward.

The subject's recognition of "its" desire, indeed even of itself as subject, is thus crucially retrospective; hence the syntax of the conjunctive synthesis, with its use of the past tense: "So that's what that was!"; "So that's what felt so intense!"; or "Oh! that was *me!*"[20] The contents of such moments of "consummation," moreover, are derived from the connections and disjunctions generated by the previous syntheses. "Just as a part of the... energy of production was transformed into energy of recording,...a part of this energy of recording is transformed into energy of consummation" (16–17/23), and a subject emerges alongside the desiring-machines to "consume," to enjoy or suffer, part of what has been produced. In the metaphysics of sovereign subjectivity, not only is that part often mistaken for the whole, but it is also attributed to the subject, when in fact the subject does no more than appropriate for itself a relatively meager portion of what has been produced and selected elsewhere. There is thus a significant ambiguity in the other formulation Deleuze and Guattari give for the conjunctive synthesis: "It's me, and so it's mine" (16/23). Here the subject in fact only arises in the consuming appropriation and consummating recognition of the results of desiring-production, yet it tends to construe itself as an autonomous entity capable of taking possession of products of the processes that in fact constitute it. The recognition that "they're me!" (in the sense that my self derives from them) succumbs to the claim that "they're mine!" (they belong to me).

This reversal of the relation between process and product, which is crucial to such misrecognition (*méconnaissance*) on the part of the subject and conducive to the illusion of sovereign subjectivity, is made possible by the earlier process/product reversal of the disjunctive synthesis, whereby only results of the suspension of the process of connective synthesis register on the body-without-organs – as differences among "finished" products. The process of connective synthesis is not just continual: this and then that, and then this, and so on; it is for that very reason equally evanescent. Desiring-production thus registers permanently in the psyche (gets stored in memory) only when it is attracted by, and its results get recorded on, the body-without-organs. At this point, what is merely a recording-surface henceforth appears to be the source of what gets recognized in the constitution of the subject in conjunctive syntheses. Finally, the subject in turn claims mastery or ownership of the body-without-organs – or of its products: consummate experience, intensities – when it is in fact merely derivative of them. The subject as product claims as its own the very process that constitutes it as subject.

Indeed, even to speak of "the" subject in the singular is in a sense to have already succumbed to the reversal and the illusions of sovereign subjectivity, for even the last of the syntheses, the conjunctive synthesis, produces a subject always different from itself on the body-without-organs. Just as much as the connective synthesis is continual (and...and...and...), and the disjunctive synthesis of recording is open-ended (or...or...or...), the conjunctive synthesis in turn generates, from the latter's vast networks of relations among organ–machines on the body-without-organs, an indefinite series of constellations or states of intense experience, each of which gets recognized and consummated *ex post facto* (or *après coup*, in Lacan's phrase) by a subject of that experience. And if this subject has

> no specific or personal identity, if it traverses the body-without-organs without destroying [the latter's] indifference [to any subjectivity], this is because it is not only a part that is peripheral to the machine, but also a part that is itself divided into parts that correspond to [the connective and disjunctive syntheses] brought about by the machine. Thus the subject consumes and consummates each of the states through which it passes, and is born of each of them anew...
>
> (41/49; translation modified)

Of course, subjects often believe themselves to have a specific and fixed identity – and so in a sense, i.e. as a result, they do. The neurotic and the pervert, as we saw, both have a fixed personal identity in which desiring-machines are locked in a specific configuration favoring either production (the pervert) or anti-production (the neurotic).

But the forces of production and anti-production also interact in other, less rigid ways to produce mobile personality-structures which remain closer to the continual, open-ended, indefinite nature of the syntheses and there-fore enjoy or suffer experience with much greater intensity.[21] As we saw, Deleuze and Guattari designate catatonia as the state of zero intensity: total breakdown; the syntheses extinguished completely: no connections, no recording, no subject.[22] It forms a kind of base-line against which to measure the forces of attraction and repulsion operating on the active body-without-organs. The paranoiac experiences the entire panoply of desiring-machines as threatening and wants to repel them, but without losing touch with them altogether (as the catatonic does). Here the forces of repulsion predominate, yet the forces of attraction are still in play: constantly repelling the desiring-machines, with no prospect of ever completely succeeding, is itself a form of intensity, especially compared to the zero-degree intensity of the full body-without-organs. The schizo, by contrast, affirms the forces of both attraction and repulsion, and takes them to the limit. Instead of being repelled or merely having their finished products registered, the connective syntheses are brought back into play and put into operation on a body-without-organs whose disjunctive syntheses multiply their ramifications indefinitely, thereby fueling the consummation of a perpetually renewed "nomadic" subject always different from itself, a kind of "permanent revolution" of psychic life. To sum up their view of schizophrenia as a process and of the subject that results from it, Deleuze and Guattari say that

> the proportions of attraction and repulsion on the body-without-organs produce, starting from zero, a series of states...and the subject is born of each state in the series, is continually reborn of the following state that determines him at a given moment, consuming–consummating all these states that cause him to be born and reborn (the lived state coming first, in relation to the subject that lives it).
>
> (20/27)

The conjunctive synthesis of consumption–consummation thus does produce "a" subject – or rather "some" subjectivity: series of lived subject-states – but without necessarily culminating in a fixed subject possessed of a specific identity.

The five paralogisms of psychoanalysis

We are now in a position to contrast the dynamics of schizophrenic subjectivity as it emerges from the regime of syntheses comprising the schizoanalytic model of the psyche with the specifics of Oedipal subjectivity as it is constructed in the nuclear family under capitalism and subsequently reinforced by psychoanalysis. As we shall see, Oedipal subjectivity involves a systematically illegitimate use of the same syntheses as underlie schizophrenic subjectivity (and perversion and paranoia, for that matter): the schizoanalytic model of psychodynamics is thus valuable not only for giving psychiatry a materialist foundation in the operations of differential repetition, but for the critique of Oedipus that it enables and performs.

In effect, everything revolves around the body-without-organs. For it is here that the productive connections of desire register as signs. Such signs, being radically polyvocal, do not (yet) mean anything, but they do introduce into the machinery of desire the potential for variation – and therefore the possibility of error, and even deceit, as well. Schizoanalysis shows the Freudian Oedipus complex to comprise a set of mistakes about the nature of desire. These mistakes are understandable, inasmuch as they reflect and indeed reinforce the apparent objective movement of reproduction in the nuclear family under capitalism, but they are serious mistakes nonetheless. Deleuze and Guattari call them "the five paralogisms of psychoanalysis," and exposing them constitutes the backbone of the internal critique of Oedipus.[23]

36

The paralogism of displacement and the critique of representation (1)

The central error psychoanalysis makes regarding the Oedipus complex is "to conclude directly from...the prohibition [against incest] the nature of what is prohibited" (114/136):

> The law tells us: You shall not marry your mother, and you shall not kill your father. And...docile subjects say to [them]selves: so that's what I wanted!
>
> (114/136)

Such is the ruse of the law prohibiting incest (and perhaps of law in general): it presents desire with a falsified image of what desire "wants" in the very act of prohibiting it. Desire is thereby trapped in a first paralogism, a classic double-bind that Deleuze and Guattari call the "paralogism of displacement": docile subjects supposedly discover what they desire at the same time that they discover they cannot have it. The law, however, Deleuze and Guattari insist, is not a natural or mechanical system, but rather a semiotic system, a system of representation. It is therefore comprised not of two terms – such as cause and effect, from the first of which one could deduce something certain about the latter – but of three terms: a signifier, a signified, and a referent, from the first two of which it is impossible to conclude anything directly about the third. They thus bring to bear the well-known poststructuralist "critique of representation," to drive a wedge between the prohibition against incest and the true nature of the desire supposedly prohibited by it.[24]

What they call the "repressing representation" is one thing: it is the signifier of the prohibition: "incest"; "Oedipus." This signifier entails or indeed generates a corresponding signified, what Deleuze and Guattari call the "displaced represented," by which they mean the distorted image of desire produced by the representation itself: the Oedipus complex. The referent, however, which Deleuze and Guattari refer to as the "repressed representative," is something else altogether: desire itself in the form it takes operating *beneath* the prohibitive system of representation in a given mode of social-production. What really gets repressed by the prohibition is thus completely different from the false image of it produced by the prohibition: desire gets *displaced* onto an erroneous signified belonging to the prohibitive system of representation rather than to desire itself. Far from being repressed by the incest prohibition, Oedipal desire is in fact produced by it (and then gets repressed by it only after the fact); the Oedipus complex, Deleuze and Guattari insist, is a "falsified apparent image that is meant to trap desire" (115/136–7).

As basic as this first – capital – mistake is to psychoanalysis, however, the mechanism of displacement does not by itself distinguish the Oedipus from any other representation of desire; to do this we will need to examine its relations to the other four psychoanalytic misunderstandings of desire.[25] According to schizoanalysis, any fixed representation – prohibitive or not – distorts the true protean nature of desire. The constitutive *ambivalence* of the body-without-organs is such that it lays desire open to distortion and capture by representation at the same time and in the same process – the registration of desire in signs – that opens it to infinite variation.[26] In this, Deleuze and Guattari are clearly indebted to Lacan, who was the first to insist that the unconscious was structured like a sign-system, i.e. like a language. But the conclusions they draw are very different: as a neo-Heideggerian existentialist, Lacan insists that the advent of semiotics in the unconscious entails the tragic loss of any direct contact between consciousness and bodily drives, as we have seen. There is thus no recourse but to resign yourself to the meaninglessness of the unconscious and "enjoy your symptom," since consciousness amounts to neurosis. Deleuze and Guattari agree that the unconscious is meaningless; indeed, for them, it does not comprise a single sign-system (e.g. language), but many. The machine-connections of the drives thus cannot ever attain "faithful" representation: the content of any representation inevitably distorts desire. Yet even though the content of representation may be unreliable, its form-of-semiosis constitutes for Deleuze and Guattari a crucial index of the extent to which a given system of representation agrees with or contravenes the dynamics of unconscious desire as understood by schizoanalysis. This criterion makes what I have called the materialist semiotics of Deleuze and Guattari a critical and even a revolutionary semiotics as well. The stance of schizoanalysis is so much more affirmative than Lacanian psychoanalysis largely because of this insistence that criteria do exist by which we can distinguish illegitimate from legitimate usage of the syntheses, and thereby evaluate the form-of-semiosis, if not the content, of systems of representation. And the psychoanalytic Oedipus can be formally distinguished as a specific betrayal of the true schizophrenic unconscious by its systematically illegitimate uses of the syntheses of desire, to which we now turn.

The paralogism of application and illegitimate use of the conjunctive synthesis

In doing so, however, it is worth noting one further advance Deleuze and Guattari make over Lacan. Like him, they recognize the importance of semiotics for understanding the unconscious. But schizoanalysis is a materialist semiotics, which in the present connection means that the nuclear family itself, as a social institution and an ensemble of material practices, is understood to constitute a system of representation just as much as do psychoanalysis and its discursive analyses of the "Oedipus complex." Indeed, for schizoanalysis, the real nuclear family is if anything a more important system of representation than are the discourse and practice of psychoanalysis, since the latter merely reinforces the "apparent objective movement" of the nuclear family as a capitalist institution:

> We have never dreamed of saying that psychoanalysis invented Oedipus. Everything points in the opposite direction: the subjects of psychoanalysis arrive already Oedipalized, they demand it, they want more....All that psychoanaly[sis does] is reinforce the movement, add a last burst of energy to the displacement of the entire unconscious.
>
> (121/144)

If Oedipal representations of desire register so forcefully on the body-without-organs and so often succeed in displacing and trapping desire in Oedipal subjectivity, it is first and foremost because that is the way desire is actually lived at the heart of the nuclear family. Yet that in no way legitimates the claims to universality made by psychoanalysis in the name of Oedipus: on the contrary, it points up the historical specificity of the nuclear family as an institution of reproduction and adds urgency to the calls made by schizo-analysis to bring psychoanalysis to the point of self-criticism and to overthrow the Oedipus in both its material and its discursive systems of representation.

Deleuze and Guattari take this argument yet one step further, for schizo-analysis is not just a materialist semiotics: it is an historical-materialist semiotics. Not only is the nuclear family as social institution the basis for Oedipalized subjects and Oedipal representations of desire (including psychoanalysis) alike, historically speaking it is only the latest in a long line of social institutions responsible for the construction of fixed subjectivities, and it is in some ways the weakest and the most abstract. Fixed subjects of all kinds arise from an illegitimate use of the conjunctive synthesis that segregates one set of subjectivities from all the others and demands that an otherwise nomadic subjectivity (resulting from legitimate conjunctive syntheses) identify only with members of that restricted set: whites rather than blacks; men rather than women; Christians rather than Jews, and so forth. Instead of the "I am everyone and anyone" of the nomadic subject, the segregated subject believes that he/she belongs to a "superior race" (103–105), identifies himself/herself as essentially different from and better than all the others from which he/she is segregated. Historically, the content or rationale for such segregation has varied considerably: totem, clan, religion, race, nation, sorority/fraternity, sports team, and so on. But the form of the illegitimate synthesis remains the same: on the basis of a segregation aligning the subject with a superior "us" versus an inferior "them," a fixed sense of identity arises that rejects as undesirable the multiform possibilities of nomadic subjectivity.

What is so striking about the nuclear family as the modern version of such segregative reproduction of subjectivity is the severity of the segregation imposed. Because capitalism so radically isolates reproduction in the private or domestic sphere from production in the public sphere, Oedipal subjects are offered no one to identify with except Mommy or Daddy. Even compared to pre-modern reproductive institutions, with their animals, ancestors, saints, gods, and so on – not to mention the rich multiplicities of schizophrenic subjectivity – the Oedipal subject occupies a terrain that is remarkably poor in objects of identification. One result is that the only remaining distinctive feature supporting identification within the family is bare gender: male or female. I shall return to this constriction of possibilities in connection with the illegitimate use of the disjunctive synthesis. For now, we will note that the segregation of the nuclear family from society drastically reduces to only two the range of subject-positions generated within it: prohibited object of desire (Mommy), on the one hand, and agent of the prohibition (Daddy), on the other. That is why Oedipal subjectivity is so abstract, so guilt-ridden, so "modern": because of its entrapment in the narrow confines of the nuclear family as a segregated institution of reproduction under capitalism. At the same time, however, it is largely because Oedipal subjectivity has been bled of all other social determinations than these that it tends to be so weak, and constantly requires shoring up from the "inside," i.e. via psychoanalytic therapy, as well as from "without," via sundry state patriotisms, ethnic racisms, religious fundamentalisms, sports fanaticisms, and so on.[27]

The capital mistake made by psychoanalysis in this connection is to interpret these fully social determinations of subjectivity (racial, political, religious, etc.) in terms of the Oedipus complex, when the opposite is the case: familial segregation is not only historically derivative of these other segregative forms, but these latter have never ceased to operate in the modern "public sphere" and they effectively overdetermine the reproduction of subjectivity delegated under capitalism to the nuclear family:

> In a word, the family is never a microcosm, [never] an autonomous figure....[It] is by nature eccentric, decentered....There is always an uncle from America; a brother who went bad; an aunt who took off with a military man; a cousin out of work, bankrupt, or a victim of the Crash; an anarchist grandfather; a grandmother in the hospital, crazy or senile....The family does not engender its own ruptures. Families are filled with gaps and transected by breaks that are not familial: the Commune, the Dreyfus Affair, religion and atheism, the Spanish Civil War, the rise of fascism, Stalinism, the Vietnam War, May '68 – all these things form complexes of the unconscious, more effective than everlasting Oedipus.
>
> (97/116)

Despite its apparent segregation from society at large, the nuclear family is not an autonomous microcosm but merely a relay for the real determinants, which for schizoanalysis are always social and historical in nature.

In fact, schizoanalysis claims not just that Oedipal familial relations are subordinate to social relations, but that they might as well have been "fabricated to meet the requirements of [the capitalist] social formation" (101/120), for reasons I will examine in Chapter 3. What is important for present purposes is that, in reducing the polyvocal nature of nomadic conjunctions and the multiplicity of real socio-historical determinants to the Oedipus complex, psychoanalytic interpretation makes a second illegitimate use of the conjunctive synthesis, which Deleuze and Guattari call "bi-univo-calization": the reduction of the real complexity of the unconscious to an expressive relation between an "everlasting" tenor that is held constant, on the one hand – the Oedipus – and on the other a vehicle – comprising all the socio-historical material – that varies substantially but for psychoanalysis enjoys no explanatory power whatsoever. Hence the tiresome, mechanically repetitive quality of psychoanalytic studies of culture and society: everything amounts to the Oedipus (for Freud), to lack, castration or the phallus (for Lacan), to some "kernel of surplus-enjoyment" (for Zizek[28]).

In the two illegitimate uses of the conjunctive synthesis, then, we have an "objective error" of social organization, as it were, compounded by an interpretive error of psychoanalytic exegesis. To the extent that social groups are organized around binary hierarchies segregating an "us" from a "them" (as they all too often are), restricted subjects are constructed via identification with a "superior race," nationality, religion, or whatever.[29] Within the nuclear family as reproductive institution, identification is even more severely restricted, while at the same time it grows increasingly abstract: it gets limited to the twin figures of the prohibitor and the prohibited, which serve as relays for various figures of the oppressor and the oppressed. Psychoanalysis then falls into the trap laid by the nuclear family as system of reproduction–representation, and commits a second paralogism, which Deleuze and Guattari call the "paralogism of application," by applying the Oedipal-triangular grid to everything, that is, by insisting on bi-univocalized interpretations that constantly reduce all the rich complexity of real social determinations to these narrow, abstract figures of the Oedipus complex: "So this is what all that means: it was your father, or it was your mother" (101/120).

The paralogism of the double-bind and illegitimate use of the disjunctive synthesis

At the same time, such Oedipalizing interpretation makes illegitimate use of the disjunctive synthesis of recording. Instead of offering an open-ended series containing manifold possibilities for identification, the nuclear family first of all restricts the possibilities to Mommy and Daddy, and then

41

imposes an exclusive choice between them: you must be either like Mommy or like Daddy: not like anybody else (your uncle from America, your unemployed cousin, your grandmother in the hospital...) and not even a little like each of Mommy and Daddy in some respects yet different in others. This is the illegitimate – that is, restrictive and exclusive – use of the disjunctive synthesis that depends directly on the segregation of the nuclear family as reproductive institution from the rest of social life and its reduction of the basis for identification to gender alone. But there are additional instances of illegitimate disjunctive synthesis comprising the Oedipus.

Indeed, to focus too narrowly on the familial Oedipus and the fixed subject-positions it constructs via identification with Daddy or Mommy would be to ignore the advances made by Lacan in the form of a linguistic or structural psychoanalysis. For Lacan argues that the Oedipus complex is concerned only apparently (i.e. in the Imaginary register) with the concrete figures of father and mother; it actually (i.e. in the Symbolic register) involves functions rather than figures or images: the functions of agent of prohibition or Law, and object of prohibition or desire. Deleuze and Guattari acknowledge the importance of Lacan's attempt to de-personalize psychoanalysis, but they argue that he did not go far enough in reducing or elevating it to a purely functional analysis. Notoriously, the phallus is impossible to strip of its associations with the male sex organ, despite Lacan's desire to construe it as purely a differentiating function; in a similar way, it is difficult to detach the "lack" that for Lacan defines human psychology in general from its associations with the "hole" or the result of castration represented by the female sex organ: images from the Imaginary register inevitably cling to the functions he wants to distinguish as purely Symbolic. Ultimately, Deleuze and Guattari argue, the familial and the structural versions of the Oedipus, as well as the Imaginary and Symbolic registers themselves, are indistinguishable. Or rather, the differences between them remain in force, but instead of being differences between distinct, stable entities, they are differences that define those entities only in relation to one another. Constitutive differences are what remain, while the distinction between entities becomes "undecidable" (81/96).[30] So instead of positing an exclusive disjunction between Imaginary and Symbolic which would enable a clear distinction to be drawn between them, Deleuze and Guattari propose an inclusive disjunction according to which Imaginary and Symbolic are different but not distinct, their differences ultimately undecidable, serving to inextricably relate rather than segregate or separate.

By contrast, insofar as the Lacanian disjunction between Imaginary and Symbolic is construed as exclusive (the Real having been declared "impossible"), it comprises another Oedipal double-bind, a third paralogism which Deleuze and Guattari refer to as the "paralogism of the double-impasse" (110/131; see also 79–81/94–6).[31] For the Oedipus complex appears to present two, and only two, possibilities: resolution or fixation. "Successful" resolution, given the specific restricted conditions of the nuclear family, means internalizing self-denial and submitting to Oedipal authority: accepting the incest-taboo entails differentiating oneself from one's parents and pursuing "Symbolic" substitutes in their place. Unsuccessful negotiation of the complex, meanwhile, means refusing the differentiating function of the castrating phallus and remaining trapped in the nuclear family and the restricted identifications it supports/inflicts. In sickness and in health, it is always Oedipus that wins: one either becomes a differentiated father-substitute and passes it on to the children in a new family, or remains an undifferentiated father-rival fixated on the old family. Either way, the possibilities are restricted to the undecidable alternative: Imaginary fixation or Symbolic resolution, neurosis or "normality."

But beneath or beyond the restricted alternatives of the Oedipal double-impasse, legitimate disjunctive syntheses ceaselessly affirm other differences; the schizo explores mobile subjectivities that are not definable in terms of absolute differentiation or undifferentiation, since each one is lived and affirmed as different. Here, again, Deleuze's materialist ontology of difference is crucial, inasmuch as it enables us to understand the patterns of repetition generating subjectivity otherwise than in terms of the binary opposition of absolute differentiation versus undifferentiation. And neither is schizophrenic subjectivity definable exclusively in terms of Mommy and Daddy, for if a schizo does identify with parental figures, it is only temporarily and as one among many polyvocal substitutes for other figures altogether: some animal, group, god, or planet having nothing to do with the Oedipal family.

Deleuze and Guattari then take the case against exclusive disjunction one step further, arguing against one of the cornerstones of Lacan's structural psychoanalysis, the binary opposition involved in what he sometimes called the "Real" difference between the sexes: the necessity of being either male or female.[32] Deleuze and Guattari categorically deny the validity of the opposition. No one is really exclusively male or female any more than they are exclusively heterosexual or homosexual; everyone is at the same time neither and both: neither in the sense of remaining irreducible to any single essence, while still entertaining elements of both, yet without combining the two into any kind of synthesis that would eliminate the differences between them. Such is the form of subjectivity produced by inclusive disjunctive synthesis.

As in the case of illegitimate conjunctive syntheses which fail to completely segregate the nuclear family, exclusive gender disjunctions even within the nuclear family ultimately fail to impose binary sexuality. The family supposedly starts with only two sexes available for identification: male and female. But that illegitimately excludes homosexuality: if we include homosexuality, the number of sexes increases to four (in alphabetical order: heterosexual female, heterosexual male, homosexual female, homosexual male). But then there are also two modes of relation – object-choice and identification – so the possibilities for sexual "identity" multiply yet again: we could distinguish male-identified homosexual females with female object-choice (butch–femme relations) from male-identified homosexual females with male object-choice (butch–butch relations); male-identified heterosexual males with female object-choice ("normal" Oedipal relations) from male-identified heterosexual females with male object-choice (a kind of "inverted" Oedipal relation), and so on. Even on this level, which still presupposes the validity of a global distinction between "male" and "female," binary sexual identity has mushroomed into multiplicity.[33]

Yet even if on what Deleuze and Guattari call the "molar" level, the level of "external" object-choice and identification, there may still be recognizable sexual identities (though clearly many more than two), on the "molecular" level sexual "identity" is comprised of a multiplicity of "internal" features (including what are sometimes called "secondary" sexual characteristics) that are not reducible to the reproductive organs alone. These may include body-hair, bone and muscle mass, breast size, propensity to aggression or passivity, to the emotional or rational, and so forth.[34] Here, too, there are no longer just two sexual identities but rather diverse ways of "being a man" which go far beyond being just "straight" or "gay," a variety of ways of being "a lesbian," say, which go far beyond being "butch" or "femme." The result, Deleuze and Guattari insist, is that there are "not one or even two, but *n* sexes" (296/352): there is no such thing as sexual identity, no such thing as heterosexuality, homosexuality, or bi-sexuality except as gross approximations – only multiplicity or what they call "trans-sexuality." It is never really a question of being either a man or a woman, either straight or gay, and so on, but of affirming a multiplicity of innumerable differences; with legitimate disjunctive syntheses, it is never a question of being either this or that, but of constantly exploring real alternatives and of (whatever one once was or is now) always becoming-otherwise: this…or this…or this…or this.

The nuclear family, by contrast, largely because as the principal reproductive institution under capitalism it is segregated from society at large, makes systematic illegitimate use of disjunctive syntheses to impose a restrictive set of ultimately untenable binary oppositions. One is either man or woman, prohibitor or prohibited; either child or parent, subjected to obeying the law or responsible for wielding it; one either resolves the Oedipal crisis or fixates on it, either blithely passing it on to one's children or endlessly repeating it on one's own; finally (with Lacan), one lives the Oedipus either as a universal existential drama of the structure of language or in the intimate theater of a personal family triangle, either as myth in general or as one of its variants. And psychoanalysis (always with the possible exception of Lacan), far from challenging or even accurately diagnosing these double-binds as such, devotes most of the energy it can muster to reinforcing and perpetuating them.

The paralogism of extrapolation and illegitimate use of the connective synthesis

Yet at the same time, schizoanalysis recognizes that psychoanalysis came very close to the heart of the matter, despite its subsequent superimposition of Oedipalizing interpretations, when it recognized the importance of libido as sexual energy in general; of drives without fixed, instinctually predetermined objects; and of free-association as an index of unconscious thought – aspects of psychoanalytic theory that get foregrounded in Melanie Klein's discussions of "partial-objects" and Lacan's of "objets petit-a." This is one reason Deleuze and Guattari refuse "to play 'take it or leave it'" with psychoanalytic theory (117/140). For example, free-association – provided it really remains free – aptly illustrates legitimate forms of connective and disjunctive synthesis: each item in the chain of associations is evaluated, not in and of itself but for the associative connections it can generate or entertain with other items, which are similarly evaluated in terms of the associative connections they entertain with others, and so on. The problem with free-association in conventional psychoanalysis is that it becomes subject to interpretation, to what Deleuze and Guattari call a process of "forcing" whereby the polyvocal connections of truly free free-association get *bi-univocalized*, reduced to the familiar litany of subjects, topics, and symbols: every woman is the mother, every aggression a parricide, anything concave or hollow a symbol of feminine "lack," anything longer than it is wide a phallic symbol. In such illegitimate use of the connective synthesis, one privileged term – the image of the mother, the name of the father, the phallus, or whatever – is detached from the chain of associations and assigned the role of general interpretant for all of them.[35] As a general rule, psychoanalysis subjects polyvocal associations to the constraints of Oedipalizing interpretation.

Deleuze and Guattari discern the same pattern of discovery and betrayal in Melanie Klein's ground-breaking work on what she called "pre-Oedipal" relations. At this early stage of development, according to Klein, the infant's experience is comprised exclusively of "part-objects": objects seen or processed solely in response to one particular drive or another, in a psyche that has not yet integrated the drives into a unified ego. The infant may, for instance, experience a "good" breast (one that gives) and a "bad" breast (which withdraws) in alternating modes of attraction and repulsion, without combining the two "versions" into a whole-object or assigning them to a global person, "the" mother. Here it is the life and death instincts which are not integrated or fused under the aegis of a unified ego or subject, but in fact any unintegrated drives can produce specific "versions" of any object, which are thereby (experienced as) part-objects. Perverts and fetishists notoriously endow their versions of ordinary objects with a peculiar erotic charge or value which is produced by the operation of certain drives outside the integration of the "normal" ego.

As the term "pre-Oedipal" itself reveals, however, part-object experience for Klein is just a stage in a process leading to a subsequent "depressive" stage where the integration of drives is achieved in or by a now-unified subject. Deleuze and Guattari do not deny that the conversion of partial-objects to whole-objects takes place: however, they insist, first of all, that such conversion is an effect of repression and representation on the body-without-organs, a capture of desire in a certain type of signifying chain, which I will examine below. They furthermore deny that the conversion to whole-objects can ever be complete, and refuse to interpret partial-objects retrospectively in terms of the Oedipus: unified subjectivity exists only as an after-effect alongside the desiring-machines, and these latter continue to make and break connections and disjunctions among partial-objects even after subjectivity arises, in ways that would therefore have to be called "an-Oedipal" rather than "pre-Oedipal."[36] Finally, and most important, they agree with Nietzsche that subjectivity at every stage of development comprises a largely subconscious struggle among competing drives for mastery of the psyche, and that it is only the temporary victory of one of them that produces the illusion of conscious mastery and unity. Far from being "pre-Oedipal" and childish, then, partial-objects for schizoanalysis register the competing claims made by disparate drives to process experience according to divergent criteria of value or what Nietzsche might call differing "perspectives." This crucial insight into the true nature of subjectivity is lost on Klein, however, since she posits a natural progression through the depressive stage culminating in an integrated ego.

This endorsement of Nietzschean perspectivism makes certain aspects of Lacanian psychoanalysis interesting to Deleuze and Guattari, for Lacan took Klein's work in a similar direction. He, too, refused to play "take it or leave it" with psychoanalytic theory: he accepts the notion of partial-objects (which he calls *objets petit-a*), but rejects the notion that they are subsequently integrated into a unified ego as the culmination of a natural process of development, as Klein had claimed. Lacan's critique of the unified ego, to which we will return in a moment, is categorical; his position on the semiotic processes supporting such an ego, however, is not so clear. Lacan tends to salvage illegitimate aspects of psychoanalytic theory – viz. the Oedipus complex itself! – by translating them into a linguistic idiom that reproduces their semiotic form (in or as the Symbolic) even while rejecting their content (as Imaginary), instead of submitting them to critique or bringing them to the point of autocritique, as Deleuze and Guattari aim to do.[37]

On Deleuze and Guattari's analysis, the illegitimate use of the connective synthesis comprises a fourth paralogism, which they call the "paralogism of extrapolation." It takes two forms. One involves the illegitimate extrapolation of global persons as complete-objects from partial-object relations;

this is the error they diagnose in the work of Melanie Klein. The other consists in extracting one particular partial-object from the flow of experience and transforming it into a specially privileged complete-object in terms of which all other partial-objects and indeed experience in general are to be evaluated or understood. This is precisely the role Lacan grants to the phallus in his linguistic version of the Oedipus complex, and the issue raised by schizoanalysis (which may finally be unresolvable) is whether the Lacanian account effectively rejects or merely reproduces the illegitimate operation involved.

For Freud, the Oedipus complex is a family drama about separating from the Mother under threat of castration (real or implied), accepting the Father's prohibitive authority, and identifying with the same-sex parent in the search for a spouse of one's own. In Lacan's translation, the Oedipus complex becomes a more broadly existential drama about the acquisition of language and the entry into a meaningful universe governed by the law of signification. Separation from the Mother means losing touch with the physical realm of bodily substance or "being" – not just the Mother's body, but one's own body and drives, along with the material environment in general – and accepting the realm of meaning and the law of signification in its place. In the Lacanian idiom, the prohibition against incest becomes the "non/nom du père": at one and the same time the Father's castrating "no" forbidding access to the Mother and the Father's name that identifies her as his wife, it furthermore designates the place the son will occupy in the Symbolic Order when he takes a substitute wife of his own, who will also bear his father's name. The play on the homonym "non/nom" is significant in that it translates or carries the interpersonal prohibition onto linguistic terrain: drawing on Lévi-Strauss's analysis of kinship terminology, Lacan insists that the woman as substantial being is lost at the same time and in the same process that the mother–wife is prohibited – when she becomes a meaning-laden linguistic construct made possible by the law of signification. The paternal signifier (or phallus) represents the double promise of plenitude of meaning and command of substance (the mother–wife), in relation to the castrated– separated subject as well as the forbidden substance from which it is separated, both of which appear lacking by comparison. One signifier has been selected from and elevated over the rest, to which it assigns meaning and measures of deficiency (castration, loss) in relation to its own plenitude. Under the aegis of the paternal signifier, the castrated subject translates the search for lost substance into a search for meaningful substitutes through signifying chains fueled by the metonymy of desire and governed by the law of signification.[38]

The Lacanian Oedipus complex is thus ultimately about substitution and the laws governing substitution. To be sure, the incest-taboo prohibits relations with parents and siblings, but it does so (as Lévi-Strauss and many other anthropologists insist) partly in order to foster relations with others who are identified within and by the laws of the Symbolic Order as possible substitutes, as future husbands or wives. Going perhaps one step beyond Lévi-Strauss's analyses of various kinship systems with their different sets of laws governing such substitutions, Lacan suggests that the name of the father founds or is homologous with the law of signification in general: To be sure, the law of signification in the Symbolic Order governs what counts as a husband or a wife and what cannot; this is the specific "content" of the incest-taboo. But the law of signification governs what counts as proper court etiquette just as surely as it governs proper courtship behavior, just as it governs what counts as a loyal subject or a capital crime, or what can count as a table or a chair. Its specific content aside, the form of the incest-taboo for Lacan is none other than the form of the law of signification itself, which governs the permissible substitutions or iterations that endow any and all experience with meaning.

This Lacanian account raises two kinds of question for schizoanalysis. First of all, does signification require the violent separation of castration and the extraction of a privileged transcendent term such as the name of the father or the phallus to make iteration in language possible, or even to make incest-free substitution in interpersonal relations desirable? Deleuze and Guattari answer no: differential repetition promotes patterns of substitution and iteration that support viable forms of signification which are not provoked by castration or governed by any transcendent law. "The possibility of living beyond the father's law, beyond all law," Deleuze and Guattari emphasize, "is perhaps the most essential possibility brought forth by…psychoanalysis" (81/97). What makes the extraction of a transcendent term – and especially a prohibitive "castrating" term – appear necessary is in fact the inertia or "innate conservatism" of instinct as psychoanalysis conceives it to begin with: in terms of mechanical repetition of the same. Except for the force of that conception, avoidance of incest could be understood to result from manifold changes wrought by differential repetition itself during the active development of the child, rather than from passive submission to castration and prohibitive law. Instead, psychoanalysis "makes us believe that real desiring-production must answer to higher formations that integrate it, subject it to transcendent laws, and make it serve a higher social and cultural production" (74/88; translation modified). Inasmuch as psychoanalysis proceeds this way from the alleged psychological necessity of castration and a transcendent law, Deleuze and Guattari pointedly conclude: "all resignations are justified in advance" (74/88).

It may well be that Lacan never wholeheartedly endorses this interpretation of desire as necessary, but merely diagnoses it as what actually prevails. But even if we were to accept the necessity (which schizoanalysis denies) of a transcendent term to govern substitution and iteration, there is no (psycho) logical reason why it could not be the mother's breast rather than the phallus or the name of the father. There are, of course, good (socio-)historical reasons to choose the name of the father and the phallus as the transcendent terms of the law: as a way of targeting patriarchy, phallocentrism, and phall-ogocentrism. But it is not clear that this is what Lacan meant to do (though he has been read this way, to great effect[39]). On the contrary, having taken relatively concrete studies of symbolic structures by Lévi-Strauss as one of his points of departure, Lacan seems to have moved increasingly toward a more formal and abstract, purely mathematical understanding of the Symbolic Order over the course of his career. I have already alluded to the difficulty of trying to expunge all socio-historical content from terms like "phallus" and "name of the father," even when the latter is called a mere "paternal metaphor" and the former is considered a pure function or signifier of absence in the Symbolic Order.

This brings us to the second kind of question schizoanalysis raises about the Lacanian account, having shown that transcendent law is not (psycho-) logically necessary: to what extent is it historically true? What historical conditions are necessary for, or indeed themselves require, the extraction of a privileged term and the imposition of a transcendent law? Conversely, and more importantly, what historical conditions make it possible to diagnose transcendent law as necessary – or unnecessary?

The answers Deleuze and Guattari provide to these questions are complicated, and will occupy most of the next chapter. For now, the short answer is that, historically speaking, Lacan's "paternal metaphor" must be considered precisely a metaphor, i.e. a substitute, for two reasons. First, in relation to the past, the father-figure of the nuclear family merely substitutes as the transcendent term governing iteration for earlier figures whose authority was, however, fully social (if not cosmic) in scope: kings, despots, gods. Second, in the present, the nuclear father-figure can finally be identified by Lacan as merely a metaphor because even his diminished role has been eclipsed in contemporary society by capital, which governs substitutions of a very different kind: those of economic exchange. What Deleuze and Guattari are able to show, as the next chapter will indicate, is that by segregating reproduction from production at large, capitalism is able both to provide an apparently transcendent term governing social relations that is completely abstract – *money* – and to continue to produce global persons as concrete, apparently unified, egos in the intimate space of the nuclear family. It is to Lacan's critique of these latter that I now return.

The unified ego, Lacan insists, is not a biological, physiological, or psychological given, but a fiction or construct based on "lack" – or, more precisely, on the impulse to disguise or deny lack. In Lacan's critique of unified subjectivity, lack has two principal aspects, corresponding roughly to what he calls the Imaginary and the Symbolic registers. The subject is first caught in a "line of fiction" during the "mirror-stage" (Lacan's version of Klein's "depressive" stage), which founds the Imaginary register. At this stage of development, the relatively uncoordinated infant perceives an apparently coordinated image of itself in a mirror or in another and older figure such as the mother, and identifies with it. And it is not only the ego that attains illusory unity and wholeness in the mirror-stage but the experience of things: the transition from partial-objects to whole-objects affects ego and things reciprocally, as it were, with things appearing increasingly complete in themselves and distinct from one another (detachable from the flux of experience) at the same time that they appear increasingly separate, as whole-objects, from the integral self. The infant assumes or is captured by this specular whole-image of itself, even though it actually lacks the self-mastery the image seems to possess. From the start, the subject is thus lacking with respect to the unified ego-image it has of itself, and the gap between subject and ego, Lacan insists, never completely closes: investing in an illusory self-identity only magnifies the distance between them.

The illusory sense of wholeness produced by Imaginary identifications in the mirror-stage is then compounded by the subject's entry into the Symbolic Order of language, within which the fledgling ego has long since been assigned a place through the *imprimatur* of a proper name. Inasmuch as the Symbolic Order is purely differential, the infant entering it loses the substantiality of its body and its drives (or loses its being, as Lacan puts it), but it also thereby gains entrance to the universe of meaning and recognition in society, through the use of the pronoun shifters "you" and "I." The speaking subject henceforth, according to Lacan, lacks access to its own body, lacks the ability to grasp or express its substantial being in the only means made available to it: differential language. Investing in an illusory plenitude of meaning only renders that inability more acute.

This sequence of development, along with the psychic structure that results from it, are sometimes represented by Lacan in a diagram called the "L-schema," a partial approximation to which is reproduced here – with the addition of a horizontal line separating the bottom and top halves of the diagram (see Figure 2.1).

S initially represents indeterminate subjectivity entertaining polyvocal relations ($\longleftarrow$------$\longrightarrow$) with partial-objects, designated by a (*objets petit-a*). But then the ego as illusory self-image (designated by a') arises from mirror-reflection in one of those objects, in the process (designated by the diagonal going from upper right to lower left, from a to a') through which Imaginary wholeness is attributed to both ego and objects and access to partial-objects occupying the domain of being is lost. And, at the culmination of the process, the illusory whole ego is reinforced by and gains access to the meaningful universe of the Symbolic Order (a double relation designated by $\longleftarrow$-----$\longrightarrow$), at the same time that the subject is split ($\$$) through its relation to the discourse of the Other, A (a relation designated by the diagonal going from lower right to upper left, from A to $\$$). Among other things, the schema is meant to indicate how deficient the ego really is, both in relation to the

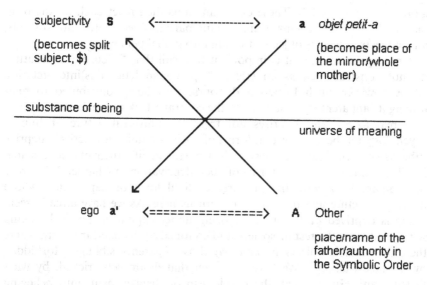

Figure 2.1 Adaptation of Lacan's "L-schema"

Imaginary image as achievement of self-mastery and in relation to the Symbolic Order as plenitude of social meaning.[40]

Yet as virulent as the Lacanian critique of the unified subject has appeared (and as much of a stir as it may have occasioned among ego-psychologists), there is an important sense in which Lacan nonetheless maintains the perspective of the ego – albeit in the form of a split subject constructed at the intersection of the Imaginary and Symbolic registers – over and against the perspective of the body and bodily desire. First of all, Deleuze and Guattari point out, there is lack only with respect to the illusions of self-mastery and meaningful plenitude, not in itself; lack is merely a secondary after-effect of the illusions of ego and meaning, not an original condition and the latter's cause and ground. This is a first reason for bisecting the Lacanian schema: nothing is lacking at the start of the process, in the top half of the schema, where indeterminate subjectivity entertains polyvocal relations with partial-objects in accordance with the legitimate use of connective syntheses.[41] Lack is instead an effect of developments leading to the bottom half of the schema, where the ego and the mother and then the father are constituted as whole-objects in the Imaginary register and assigned stable roles and fixed meanings in the Symbolic Order. This represents an illegitimate use of connective syntheses, Deleuze and Guattari insist, inasmuch as the syntheses are "global and specific" rather than partial and non-specific: "In the [former], desire at the same time receives a fixed subject, an ego specified according to sex, and complete objects defined as global persons" (70/83). These determinations then react back on the original top half of the schema, transforming partial-objects into whole-objects, and subjects as well as objects of desire into global persons.

Once again, though, it is important to recall that Deleuze and Guattari do not construe lack as an effect of psychoanalytic (mis)interpretation alone, however much Lacanian discourse may have contributed to reinforcing its apparent inevitability. On the contrary, lack is a real after-effect of very real forces, and it arises not from the universal nature of human psychology but because certain forms of social organization actively deprive subjects of their objects of desire, their means of life, their objective being. I will examine a variety of forms of such deprivation in Chapter 3, in order to compare them with the properly Oedipal form of deprivation whose internal structure and dynamics concern us here. As we have already seen, desire is deprived of its objective being under capitalism partly by being segregated from the rest of society and confined to the nuclear family, where the only available objects are *precisely* those – parents, siblings – forbidden by the incest-taboo.[42] We have also seen that desire gets tricked, by what Deleuze and Guattari call the paralogism of displacement, into believing incorrectly that it desires what is taboo, because of the existence of the taboo itself. Indeed, following Lévi-Strauss and Lacan, Deleuze and Guattari conclude that the taboo itself is responsible for the constitution of global persons, which come into being only in the very act of being prohibited.[43] No partial-objects, no breast, no connections between sex-organs, are taboo in and of themselves, only when they are seen as "belonging" to whole-objects and to the "wrong" global persons.

The incest-taboo is thus itself an illegitimate use of the connective synthesis that simultaneously "refer[s] the objects of desire to global persons [and] desire to a specific subject" (72/85), so that "partial-objects now seem to be taken from [and assigned to] people, rather than from the non-personal flows" of legitimate connective synthesis (71/85). And it is the segregated nuclear family, of all reproductive institutions, that does the most to cut its subjects off from all the non-personal flows traversing society at large and to focus desire exclusively and precisely on those whom the prohibition constitutes as global persons – which is why, Deleuze and Guattari maintain, the Oedipus is lived as a complex only under capitalism, even though the incest-taboo itself is in a sense universal. Over-investment in the delusory unified ego (*a'*) and in the internalization of Symbolic authority (*A*) are never stronger than when the formative subject is effectively isolated from other people and society at large, as it is in the nuclear family under capitalism. A second reason to bisect the Lacanian schema is thus to highlight the specificity of capitalist subjectivity and suggest that the schema's relevance may be historical as much as or more than it is psychological.

But there is a third and far more important reason for bisecting the

L-schema; it involves the Symbolic and Imaginary diagonals and their impact on the nature of the relations mapped in the top half of the diagram. We mentioned above that Lacan's Symbolic and Imaginary form an illegitimately exclusive disjunction (of the closed form: *either* this *or* that) because of his exclusion of the Real, because he declares the real to be "impossible" (27/35). But the Real can be impossible only from the perspective of consciousness. Insofar as consciousness is defined linguistically, as purely differential, and the Real is defined correlatively as pure substantiality, the Real is indeed impossible – for consciousness. But it cannot be impossible for life. From the perspective of living beings, the Real is not only not impossible, it is in fact absolutely necessary. This is the fundamental difference separating Deleuze and Guattari from Lacan: he (for perfectly understandable pragmatic reasons: as a training analyst) takes the perspective of consciousness, and the talking cure; they, following Marx and Nietzsche, take the perspective of life, and the production of life. From this perspective, the original top half of the schema (the relation designated by <----> represents simply the desiring-production of the Real, inasmuch as "the objective being of desire is the Real in and of itself" (26–7/34). Thus

> Lacan's admirable theory of desire appears to have two poles: one related to "the object small-a" as a desiring-machine, which defines desire in terms of a real production...and the other related to the "great Other" as a signifier, which reintroduces...[the] notion of lack.
> (27n./34n.)

It is the productive–constitutive relation of desire to the Real that always forms the point of departure for schizoanalysis, against which to measure the superimposition of lack by social forces. (And these social forces do not always amount to the Oedipus but rather vary historically, as we shall see in the next chapter.) Several important consequences follow.

For one thing, the partial-objects' relations constitutive of the Real are not just inevitable, as I suggested above, but fundamental: even if they are not always accessible to consciousness and never fully or accurately attain representation, the operations of the connective synthesis of production form the basis of human existence for schizoanalysis (in much the same way that will-to-power does for Nietzsche[44]). The productive relations linking desire with the Real are not impossible or lacking: it is rather consciousness that is incomplete or lacking or impossible with respect to them. Desire actively produces the Real; consciousness merely re-constructs it in representations, and it is these representations that are lacking with respect to the activity of desiring-production.

Deleuze and Guattari therefore insist, for another thing, on what they call the "coextension of humankind and nature" (107/128; translation modified) whereby "Nature = Industry [and] Nature = History" (25/32):

beneath consciousness, fixed subjectivity and complete-object representations, desiring-production involves direct connections between nature as a complex of myriad partial-object relations and humankind as a complex of ever-evolving productive activities. Nature comprises nothing less than the natural body of humankind, on this view, while humankind consists of nothing more than an exceptionally productive and (for better or for worse) prolific element of nature.[45]

And inasmuch as industry = nature = history, finally, the true subject of that history – and of universal history, to the extent that it ends up freeing schizophrenia from its last constraints, those of capitalism – is neither the proletariat (as in "workers of the world unite") nor the ego (as in "where the id was, there ego shall be"): it is none other than the unconscious, the unconscious as active, productive life-force, as Nietzschean will-to-power. "The coextension of humankind and nature," according to Deleuze and Guattari, thus comprises

> a circular movement by which the unconscious, always remaining subject, produces and reproduces itself....The organized body is the *object* of reproduction by generation...not its *subject*....Sexuality is not a means in the service of generation; rather, the generation of bodies is in the service of sexuality as an autoproduction of the unconscious....[T]he unconscious has always been [an-Oedipal], an orphan – that is, it has engendered itself in the identity of nature and humankind, of the world and humankind...
>
> (107–8/128; emphases added, translation modified)

Such a view of history warrants and even expands the importance schizoanalysis ascribes to criteria (modeled, as we saw, on those of Kant) that are immanent to the unconscious – the legitimate syntheses of production, recording, and consumption–consummation – by which it diagnoses the mistakes committed in the name of Oedipus: the systematic illegitimate uses of the three syntheses embodied in modern capitalist social organization and practices as well as in discourse, in the paralogisms of psychoanalysis itself. Succeeding chapters will expand on this view of history, examining different social formations to show, among other things, how schizophrenia finally emerges under capitalism as the potential for freeing desire from capture in and by systems of representation of all kinds.

The paralogism of the afterward and the critique of representation (2)

Before that, however, we should consider the fifth paralogism diagnosed by schizoanalysis, the last recourse of a psychoanalysis desperate to save some semblance of relevance in the face of socio-historical critique (which started as early as the second generation of psychoanalysts, with Otto Fenichel and Reich): the "paralogism of the afterward" (129/153–4, 99/118–19). The importance of real social and historical factors in psychic life is finally granted, on this line of argument, but only insofar as they are understood to come after the familial factors, which form Oedipal subjectivity first during childhood: "the child is father to the man," as the saying goes. Real social relations are thereby construed merely as so many "sublimations" of Oedipal relations, which are supposed to be primary (as well as universal).

It should be clear that this last paralogism incorporates elements of the previous four, while making systematic illegitimate use of all three syntheses. For it presupposes that the productive synthesis makes specific whole-object connections to global persons in the family alone instead of general partial-object connections to the natural and social environment at large; that the conjunctive synthesis first constructs subjects within a segregated field of restricted identifications instead of from the entire field of social relations; and that the disjunctive synthesis, positing a closed either/or alternative, effectively excludes society altogether from the enclosure of the nuclear family. But the family is not separate, not an autonomous and self-contained microcosm.[46] The family is a social institution, and the nuclear family is, in fact, a capitalist institution. And to it is *delegated* the function of reproduction under capitalism as an apparently separate institution so that social-production can develop and continually revolutionize itself without regard for the reproduction of subjects and the direct management of their desire.

Such delegation explains why the family can appear to be a microcosm when really it is not; why familially constructed subjects often seem, on the one hand, so ill-suited to the specific content-requirements of social-production at any given moment of its development; why, on the other hand, the family's degree of abstraction as an apparently separate reproductive institution produces subjects perfectly suited formally to a system of social-production in constant flux. For what they learn in the nuclear family is simply to submit, as good docile subjects, to prohibitive authority – the father, the boss, capital in general – and relinquish until later, as good ascetic subjects, their access to the objects of desire and their objective being – the mother, the goods they produce, the natural environment as a whole. But that is all they need to learn: the content-requirements of social-production, as capitalism "continually revolutionizes the means of production," change too fast for the family to play much of a role in job training, for example, just as fashion and life-style fads change too fast for parents to play an adequate role in consumer training. What the Oedipal family-machine produces is just enough: obedient ascetic subjects programmed to accept the mediation of capital between their productive life-activity and their own enjoyment of it, who will work for an internalized prohibitive authority and defer gratification until the day they die, the day after retiring. Far from being autonomous, much less originary, fundamental, or universal, the

Oedipus complex of the nuclear family appears as though it had been "fabricated to meet the requirements of...[the capitalist] social formation" (101/120), from which it in fact derives by delegation.[47] And to challenge or rebel against such Oedipally constituted authority would amount to committing incest! The Oedipal machine, to the extent that it works, effectively straight-jackets desire.

Hence the importance of the critique of representation to the schizoanalytic critique of Oedipus: in delegating the formation of desire to the nuclear family as system of reproduction-representation, capitalism manages to trap desiring-production in a deceptive and misleading image of itself, the familial content of which is mostly irrelevant, even while the form of that desiring-production ultimately echoes and reinforces precisely the kind of repression exercised by capitalist social-production itself, as we have just seen.

> *It is in one and the same movement that the repressive social-production is replaced by the repressing family, and that the latter offers a displaced image of desiring-production that represents the repressed as incestuous familial drives.*
>
> (119/142)

Desiring-production and social-production are thus, in a *descriptive* sense, one and the same process, inasmuch as schizoanalysis sees no need and no room to posit any independent universal formation of desire such as Oedipus intervening between one and the other: "*social-production is purely and simply desiring-production itself under determinate conditions*" (29/36).

Yet, in a *critical* sense, desiring-production and social-production are different, inasmuch as schizoanalysis enables and expects us to judge any historical organization of social-production according to the immanent criteria provided by desiring-production itself, and thereby exposes "the repression that the social machine exercises on desiring-machines" (54/63):

> From the very beginning of this study, we have maintained both that social-production and desiring-production are one and the same, and that they have differing regimes, with the result that a social form of production exercises an essential repression of desiring-production, and also that desiring-production – "real" desire – is potentially capable of demolishing the social form.
>
> (116/138)

Such a distinction is made possible by the constitutive ambivalence of the disjunctive synthesis of recording on the body-without-organs, as Deleuze and Guattari construe it. Desire registers in signs on the body-without-

56

organs, as we saw, when primal repression (*refoulement originaire*) caused by anti-production suspends the activity of connective synthesis. As a result, desire is free to diversify through the network of sign-relations, but it can also become trapped in fixed representations deriving from and promulgating social repression (*répression*).

Delegation of social repression under capitalism to the nuclear family thus makes it appear as if there were an autonomous "psychic" repression originating in the Oedipus complex, which would only *afterward* get extended to "social repression" in society at large, through processes of sublimation and transference. But here is where the political implications of the Oedipal (mis)representation of desire become clear, for "if psychic repression did bear on incestuous desires," Deleuze and Guattari explain, "it would gain a certain independence and primacy...in relation to social repression" (113/135). And, as they go on to say, accepting this primacy would constitute a "justification for psychic repression – a justification that makes psychic repression move into the foreground and no longer considers the problem of social repression anything more than secondary" (117/139). If "psychic" repression did truly target incestuous desires, it would be justified by the natural necessity of the incest-taboo, and social repression could be seen as a mere extension or "sublimation" of that natural necessity for the sake of higher civilization (as Freud claims). But such is not the case. Hence the importance of having three terms rather than two, to foil the ruses of representation and refute the Oedipal apology for repression. Psychoanalysis considers psychic repression in the Oedipus complex to be primary and universal, and social repression to be secondary and inevitable. Schizoanalysis, by contrast, ascribes the potential for both psychic and social repression to the registration of desire on the body-without-organs in the first place, due to the primal repression occasioned by anti-production (*refoulement originaire*).[48] It is thus able to reverse the causal order proposed by psychoanalysis and show that "psychic repression is a means in the service of social repression" (119/142), thereby delegitimizing and making it possible to historicize repression. Identifying the Oedipus complex as the form of social repression belonging to capitalism in particular, by thoroughly historicizing modes of repression in general is precisely the aim of the external critique of Oedipus, which we examine in Chapter 3.

3

SOCIAL-PRODUCTION AND THE EXTERNAL CRITIQUE OF OEDIPUS

The central function of Chapter Three of *Anti-Oedipus* is to historicize social-production's repression of desiring-production, to show that Oedipus is the specifically capitalist mode of such repression by contrasting it with other modes. The account which Deleuze and Guattari provide of three modes of social-production – savagery, despotism, capitalism [1] – is best understood not as a *history* of modes of social-production but as a *genealogy* of the Oedipus. Genealogy, in the sense of the term Foucault derives from Nietzsche, is based on the premiss that historical institutions and other features of social organization evolve not smoothly and continuously, gradually developing their potential through time, but *discontinuously*, and must be understood in terms of difference rather than continuity, as one social formation appropriates and abruptly reconfigures an older institution or revives various features of extant social organization by selectively recombining them to suit its own purposes. As Deleuze and Guattari put it, "the events that restore a thing to life [in a given form of social organization] are not the same as those that gave rise to it in the first place" (261/311). The Oedipus did not arise at the dawn of civilization (with the murder of the father in the primal horde) and evolve smoothly through Greek and Elizabethan tragedy into its modern nuclear form, as psychoanalytic legend would have it. The third chapter of *Anti-Oedipus* shows on the contrary that the modern Oedipus was cobbled together out of elements from previous social formations, in which they had very different roles to play.

Genealogical analysis will thus foreground the *differences* between Oedipal reproduction and other forms of social reproduction, revealing how unlike savage and despotic repression modern Oedipal repression actually is.[2] Indeed, Chapter Three will demonstrate that the Oedipus is specific to capitalism even though the incest-taboo, upon which it appears to be predicated, is universal. On the basis of the specific difference of capitalist reproduction such a genealogy will then show where the Oedipus came from – that is to say: where the bits and pieces of older forms of social repression came from, that the Oedipus assembles into its own distinctive repressive apparatus[3] – and why such a reproductive apparatus so perfectly suits the requirements of

58

capitalist social-production. At the same time, Deleuze and Guattari's analysis of capitalist production itself will show how it fosters schizophrenia, and thus explain why schizophrenia becomes a general and pervasive tendency of capitalist society despite the counter-tendency of the Oedipus to trap free-form desire in its familial system of reproduction-representation.

The requirements, procedures, and results of genealogical analysis are quite unlike those of historiographical narrative. In Chapter Three, Deleuze and Guattari do not intend to account historically for the emergence of capitalism from older social forms, nor do they pretend to represent concretely any formerly or actually extant society. A genealogy of the Oedipus requires the reconstruction of historical modes of social-production only as "ideal-types," logical permutations of basic social organization, as shown in Figure 3.1. Although their typology loosely resembles that developed by the American anthropologist Charles Morgan – and borrowed by Engels in *The Origin of the Family, Private Property, and the State* (1972) – it is in fact based primarily on the interplay of two categories derived from Nietzsche and Marx, respectively: power and economics.

The first thing to note about this semantic system, or logical *combinatoire*, is that Deleuze and Guattari consider power to be a negative category and economics to be a positive one, for reasons that will become clearer in the analysis that follows.[4]

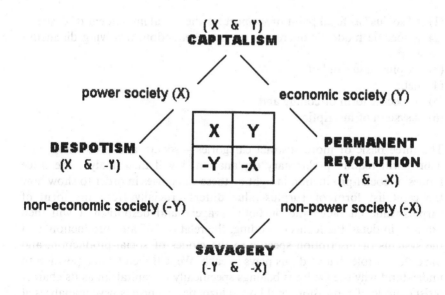

Figure 3.1 Typology of basic social organization

59

Briefly, savagery in this scheme represents something like "primitive communism," a pre-caste, pre-class form of social organization where power is diffused throughout the community rather than concentrated in any one group or individual.[5] Yet because of the absence of economics, savagery is also the social form most harshly governed by exacting codes of conduct, belief, and meaning. Under despotism, by contrast, differential codes of conduct, belief, and meaning are promulgated precisely in order to establish caste divisions and hierarchy, and are bent to the service of overt political power and direct imperial domination un-alleviated by the freedoms that become possible in economic society. Despotism thus represents the worst of both worlds, in Deleuze and Guattari's view: it is power society *par excellence*, and not economic. Capitalism, finally, is characterized by power *and* economics, which conflict with one another: the ceaselessly enhanced productivity of the capitalist economy could contribute to the general enrichment of human life-activity, but because of the capitalist power-structure it gets appropriated privately and/or devoted ascetically to increasing production for its own sake, instead. Capitalism, for schizoanalysis, is an economic society that has yet to shed its power component; the fourth term of the *combinatoire* (economics without power), which I have called "permanent revolution," appears only on its horizon, as the end of universal history.[6]

Modes of social-production, as Deleuze and Guattari understand them, are not, however, reducible to the interplay of economics and power alone; even as ideal types they are far more complex than that. Social organization and repression in each mode of social-production also involve:

(1) a "socius" as focal point or support for the social investment of desire
(2) a specific mode of operation of anti-production, involving distinctive forms of
(3) surplus-value and of
(4) debt
(5) a specific form of coding and
(6) a system of inscription.

The three basic or more abstract categories – socius, anti-production, and debt – will require preliminary explanation. I will then analyze the three modes of social-production in light of these categories in order to show how the capitalist form of surplus-value differs crucially from the form of surplus-value characteristic of both savagery and despotism. I will then examine in detail the forms of coding, the relations of anti-production, and the systems of inscription specific to the modes of social-production, and the different role that Oedipus plays in each. We will then be in a position to understand why the Oedipus belongs specifically to capitalism as its characteristic mode of repression, and how schizoanalysis brings psychoanalysis at last to the point of autocritique.

Social-production in general

Just as desiring-production is organized on the body-without-organs, social-production is organized on what Deleuze and Guattari call the "socius": the earth for savagery, the despot for barbarism, capital for capitalism.[7] It is not only the socius, as the social focal-point for the investment of productive desire, that varies historically: so does the very nature of the relationship between desiring-production and social-production.[8] In savagery, desire is bound so tightly to the socius that the organization of social-production almost completely determines the organization of desiring-production, as we shall see. Only under capitalism, partly because of its segregation of reproduction from production at large, does the organization of desiring-production become significantly different from the organization of social-production on the socius, thus allowing the body-without-organs to emerge from more or less complete determination by social-production. This is why Deleuze and Guattari say that the body-without-organs appears as such only *at the end* of history[9]: until capitalism, the body-without-organs is too powerfully over-determined by the socius to operate independently or appear in its own right.

Anti-production plays a central role in organizing social-production on the socius, just as it does with desiring-production on the body-without-organs. Indeed, like the term "desiring-machines," the concept of anti-production provides for schizoanalysis a crucial link between the realms of desiring-production and social-production. As we saw, anti-production on the body-without-organs designates what Freud and Lacan called "primal" repression (*refoulement originaire*): the advent of a process of recording in the human psyche, involving repetition, memory, representation, the formation of an unconscious. In the realm of desiring-production considered in and of itself (i.e. abstractly), the recording process is *ambivalent*: the forces of anti-production free desiring-production from strict instinctual determinism by suspending organ–machine connections, but they also make it susceptible to capture in systems of representation, as we saw in Chapter 2. We can now add this: it is consideration of the relations of social-production and anti-production that enables us to evaluate the results of the recording process, inasmuch as these relations generate the systems of representation that capture and tie desire to the socius in the institution of social organization. For such systems can either contravene or confirm the dynamics of desiring-production. And it is one of the distinctive traits of the capitalist mode of anti-production–social-production that it raises the ambivalence of the recording process to a maximum, by sponsoring both decoding and recoding.

This social sense of anti-production is derived in large part from Bataille's notion of *dépense* or expenditure. Actually, expenditure already possesses in Bataille himself both psychological and anthropological dimensions, but it is primarily the latter that will concern us here, for it provides a devastating Nietzschean critique of bourgeois political economy and utilitarian philosophy that crucially supplements that of Marx within the schizoanalytic perspective. Bataille's insights are so important that, had he not existed, schizoanalysis would have had to invent them. No society, Bataille insists, really organizes itself around needs and the production of use-values to meet needs – as necessary as such production may be to all forms of social life. Rather, social organization is always based on the expenditure of excess, and productive activity derives its meaning and purpose from such expenditure, not the other way around. Ultimately, Bataille argues, the excess to be expended derives from the astronomical amount of heat and light energy our planet receives from the sun. Various life-forms and various social forms have different ways of embodying, appropriating, organizing, concentrating, and expending their part of the excess energy-flows transiting the planet; but in all cases it is the acts of expenditure that exercise predominant influence on the life-activity of the species or social formation. This single insight provides critical correctives for three of the perspectives on which Deleuze and Guattari draw substantially in *Anti-Oedipus*.

First of all, it confirms their critique of the metaphysics of lack that has plagued Western philosophy and psychology from Plato to Lacan:

> Desire does not lack anything....[For] the objective being of desire is the Real in and of itself....Desire is not bolstered by needs, but rather the contrary; needs are derived from desire: they are counter-products within the real that desire produces. Lack is a countereffect of desire; it is deposited, distributed, vacuolized within [the] real...[when social] organization deprives desire of its objective being.
>
> (26–7/34–5)

Desire is not based on some primordial lack; nor does it derive from needs: it is instead socially organized anti-production that superimposes needs and lack on productive desire. Without the application of this corrective to psychoanalysis (and Western psychology in general), as Deleuze and Guattari put it, "all resignations are justified in advance" (74/88). The point of comparing various modes of social-production is to understand the conditions under which, and the different ways in which, anti-production introjects needs and/or lack into desiring-production.

Second, the schizoanalytic concept of anti-production introduces the issue of power into what Marx referred to as the dialectic of the "forces and relations of production." For Marx, the forces of production are always primary, even if the relations of production determine the form which production takes in a given society. All social activity not related to production in the Marxist framework tends to be relegated to the rather amorphous sphere of "reproduction."[10] For schizoanalysis, the forces of production remain important, and maintain their own autonomous dynamism as a locus and expression of desire, but (in line with Bataille) they are given form and purpose by the relations of *anti*-production. It is these relations of anti-production that organize the social expenditure of surplus in ways that either inhibit or foster the institution of power relations of various kinds. To the familiar Marxist dualisms, then, schizoanalysis adds extra terms: the dialectic of forces and relations of production becomes the interplay of forces and relations of production *and* forces and relations of anti-production; the alternative between the sphere of production or the sphere of reproduction broadens to include the sphere of anti-production.[11]

Finally, anti-production as the organization of matter- and energy-flows on the socius provides a crucial corrective to what Deleuze and Guattari call the "exchangism" of Lévi-Strauss. In fact, the concept of the socius provides a materialist basis for what Lévi-Strauss called the "symbolic order" – that is, for the codes and the systems of inscription that organize desire socially in the different modes of social-production. As Lévi-Strauss has shown, kinship terminology and myths organize desire (conduct, belief, meaning) according to the codes of a symbolic order – as do the legal codes promulgated by despots to govern the subordinate peoples of their empires, and the laws governing the sale of labor and other commodities, for example, in very different forms of symbolic order. Social coding on the socius for Deleuze and Guattari organizes bodies, practices, and objects as well as symbols and words, as it does for Lévi-Strauss. But for the founder of structuralism, social organization is ultimately everywhere the same, and always amounts to systems of *exchange* – whether of women, of words and stories, of prestige objects, or of ordinary goods. For Deleuze and Guattari, by contrast, as Chapter Three of *Anti-Oedipus* is meant to show, social organization is *not* everywhere the same: forms of coding and systems of inscription differ significantly among the three ideal-type modes of social-production they analyze, in part because desire gets organized or inscribed on the type of socius specific to each mode of social-production (as indicated above): the earth, the despot, capital. And, even more importantly, symbolic order everywhere is ultimately based not on exchange but on *debt* – which itself takes diverse forms in the different modes of social-production, as we shall see. In line with the arguments subordinating identity to difference in *Difference and Repetition*, Deleuze and Guattari consider the exchange of equivalents to be a subsidiary, and mostly illusory or mystifying, form of debt – which is a relation not of equivalence but of inequality, difference, or force.[12]

It may seem perplexing to have passed so quickly from the notion of "excess" in Bataille to that of "debt" in schizoanalysis. But the importance of the latter notion for analyzing different types of power relation will become clear in a moment. For now it may help to recall that anti-production is, in the social as well as the psychological realm, simply a transformation of productive energy or force whereby "a full body [here the socius] falls back on the economy that it appropriates" (248/295): it is the conversion of a portion of the superabundant forces of production into a counter-force that absorbs, distributes, or consumes already-produced products in the name of a creditor to whom a debt is owed. Of course the debt collectively owed to the earth in savagery is quite unlike the debt subordinate peoples owe the despot in despotism, which is again quite unlike the debt owed to capital under capitalism. Indeed, more important than the figure to whom the debt is nominally owed is the *system of anti-production* the debt sustains, for the social management of excess as debt is its primary *raison d'être*: you never pay capital itself, but a bank; never a god or king, but a priest or functionary; never the earth itself, but a shaman or ancestor. Debt is thus the general name under which relations of social obligation are enforced by anti-production; it is the principal means by which "lack...is deposited, distributed, vacuolized into [the] real" (27/34). Now what anti-production always precludes, as we shall see, is the direct appropriation and complete and immediate enjoyment of the fruits of production; and what it institutes is a variety of regimes always based on deferral, on the separation of productive force from what it can produce or already has produced, on the accumulation of reserves, the constitution and maintenance of extensive social organization, and – in certain forms under certain conditions, e.g. Oedipal guilt in the nuclear family – on thoroughgoing self-denial: asceticism. Anti-production as the controlled expenditure of excess is thus for schizoanalysis co-terminous with the process of organizing social relations in systems of debt of various kinds.

Forms of surplus-value and coding

A mode of social-production/anti-production comprises a specific form of organization for flows of matter and energy. Ultimately, there are two ways such organization can be accomplished: qualitatively or quantitatively, symbolically or economically.[13] Savagery and despotism are organized symbolically, via codes and over-codes, while capitalism is organized economically, via axioms.

The system of anti-production in savagery involves, in brief, the temporary accumulation of a surplus of specific goods – cattle, yams, or cowry shells, for instance – goods that the tribe collectively deems to be of special value or significance. Deleuze and Guattari call this a "surplus-value of code" because social codes determine what is of value and therefore worth accumulating. Extensive accumulation, however, is explicitly prohibited and actively prevented: ritual orgies of waste and expenditure (such as northwest Native American *potlatch*) prevent accumulation by obliging each clan to maintain its proper place in the symbolic order by either destroying or dispersing accumulated goods when its turn comes. Debt within the savage system of anti-production is thus sporadic and reciprocal, remains immanent to the kinship system of blood-lineages and marriage-alliances comprising savage social organization, and functions to prevent power from accruing to any one family or clan.[14]

Anti-production serves precisely the opposite function in the power structure of despotism: instead of a patchwork of debts and responsibilities following the network of lineages and alliances, all obligations now focus directly on the despot himself, transforming the sporadic and reciprocal relations of savage anti-production into an infinite and uni-directional debt. This transformation has several consequences. For one thing, inasmuch as the despot sets himself up as the sole agent of anti-production over the peoples he subordinates, he becomes the target/object of universal envy: his transcendent position of power is thus inherently paranoid. It will then become possible to contrast the paranoia characteristic of despotism with the perversion characteristic of savagery, but also with the neuroses of the nuclear family and the schizophrenia of capitalism. More important for now is the impact that the infinite and uni-directional form of despotic debt has on the means of payment and on the shape of symbolic order itself.

For despotic tribute is not payable in the various locally coded "currencies" of the despot's subject-peoples: objects of special significance to this or that group mean nothing to the despot; they are of no value outside the group. Instead, *one* single representative of value – gold – becomes the privileged signifier of universal value, and this "over-coded" form of surplus-value – expressing not local coding but a transcendent law and an *imposed standard* of value – flows continually into the bottomless coffers of the despot. From what had been a network of reciprocally constituting (Saussure would say "purely differential") relations instituting and reflecting collective agreement, one privileged term has been extracted and superimposed as the measure and guarantor of imperial value. Here, then, is a first answer to the questions raised in Chapter 2 about the Lacanian perspective as to the historical conditions which support or require the extraction of a privileged term and the imposition of a transcendent law: the "psychological" (or psycho-linguistic) function Lacan assigns (universally) to the phallus is in fact a feature of power society and its process of over-coding, not of coding (or of language) per se; it originates in the realm of social-production, not that of desiring-production; and it governs in the name of the despot, not in the name of the father. Only later, under capitalism, does it migrate into the nuclear family and govern the Oedipus complex in the father's name, as we shall see.[15]

For now, it is important to note that money – which arises, Deleuze and Guattari remind us, from imperial tribute as a means of paying debt, not from barter as a means of commercial exchange[16] – as tribute represents the first great deterritorialization of codes and meaning by abstract value: value is evacuated from meaningful objects and accrues instead to gold or money as universal equivalent. Under despotism, however, money is still an *imposed* standard of value; it is still a "foreign currency" to the local symbolic orders of the peoples who are bound to pay it. Tribute money is not yet the "common currency" of commercial money integrating the whole of market society economically, but a sign of political subordination; the abstract value of tribute money is not yet exchange-value, but debt-value, as it were. Money does not yet mediate voluntary contractual relations between (formally) equal parties, does not yet beget money all by itself, as it will under capitalism: it has to be extracted by force. So, even though it is paid in money, despotic tribute nonetheless remains a *surplus-value of code* – and specifically of the over-codes that enforce and reflect the political dominance characteristic of the imperial power-structure. (This is the principal reason why, even today, taxes – the modern form of tribute – inspire revolt as a palpable instance of political oppression, while profits do not.) Despotic anti-production transforms the patchwork of short-lived debts and obligations immanent to and constitutive of savage social organization into an infinite debt owed to the transcendent figure of the despot, who superimposes a new hierarchical form of social organization "from on high," as Deleuze and Guattari put it. But social-production is still organized in terms of local codes and imperial over-codes, so despotic surplus-value remains a surplus-value of code.[17]

What sets capitalism apart from the other modes of social-production, which code and over-code value, is that its social organization is based on the process of *axiomatization*. Symbolic codes and over-codes reflect or govern qualitative similarities among significant entities; symbolic social organization depends on regulating the relations among already-coded elements, as when social standing in savagery is associated customarily with the expenditure (*dépense*), the destruction or distribution, of items designated by the local code as prestige goods. The inter-relation of such flows is crucially indirect, inasmuch as it depends on custom – on a symbolic system of conduct, meaning, and belief. Axioms, by contrast, directly join together heterogeneous flows of matter or energy that have been quantified. Axiomatization not only does not depend on meaning, belief, and custom, but actively defies and subverts them, giving capitalism its distinctive dynamism and modernism. Quantified flows under capitalism get conjoined solely on the estimation that this or that conjunction will produce surplus-value; such estimation involves economic calculation rather than belief: symbolic meaning has nothing to do with it. And the conjunction is direct, completely unmediated by codes; indeed, the qualities attributable to axiomatized flows *arise from* the conjunction itself, rather than pre-existing it: in commodity-production and consumption, the qualities of the product ("use-values"), as well as the qualities with which the consumer is endowed by consuming it ("taste"), and also the qualities of the labor-power ("skills") and of the capital invested in machinery ("technologies") required to produce it – *all* depend on the conjunctions effected beforehand in the market via the medium of money as abstract universal equivalent.[18]

Inasmuch as the market is its basic institution and commercial money its common currency, then, capitalism substitutes a quantitative calculus based on axioms for the qualitative codes and over-codes that organized social life in previous formations. Social relations in a coded symbolic order are qualitative and significant: women in savage society, for example, are carefully named and highly valued as the source of life itself and the very cornerstone of meta-familial social relations in a kinship system fully charged with symbolic meanings. Much the same can be said of labor relations in an over-coded symbolic order, to take another example, for even when surplus-value derives from surplus-labor, as it usually does in despotism, the surplus-labor commanded by the transcendent law of the despot remains qualitatively distinct from the labor providing for the laborer's own subsistence, to the point that it may even occur at a different time and in a different place: over-coding retains and enforces a qualitative and fully meaningful distinction between the two kinds of labor. Indeed, all the resources of discourse and symbolic culture (notably those of religion) are mobilized precisely to endow the distinction with meaning and make it "believable" in the strong sense of the term.

Axiomatic social organization under capitalism, by contrast, is quantitative and strictly meaningless: nameless workers (regardless of gender) are valued only as abstractly quantified amounts of labor-power on the market, and no qualitative distinction between labor and surplus-labor any longer exists. (Even the quantitative difference between the two grows increasingly difficult to measure, much less directly perceive, and this contributes considerably to the capitalist mystification of this source of surplus-value.) The original and still fundamental capitalist axiom, as I have said, conjoins deterritorialized and quantified flows of liquid wealth – monetary wealth no longer embodied in landed property – with deterritorialized flows of "free" labor – workers no longer tied to specific means of production who therefore have no means to sustain life other than by the sale of their labor-power.[19] And in its perpetual search for new sources of profit, capitalism continually axiomatizes other qualitatively dissimilar resource-flows, transforming them into quantitatively exchangeable commodities on the market: flows of raw materials and labor skills, to be sure, but also of scientific knowledge, consumer preferences, and so on.[20]

Deleuze and Guattari will thus call capitalist surplus-value a *surplus-value of flow*, rather than of codes or over-codes: it arises as the quantitative differential between the flow of money invested in factors of production (including the production of consumption) – labor, materials, technology (and marketing) – and the flow of money returning at the end of the production–consumption cycle.[21] It matters not at all *what* (qualitatively) is produced, only *that* production occurs and surplus-value is realized. Social-production is no longer organized locally in support of a network of mobile debt-relations, nor is it organized hierarchically by and for the sake of a transcendent instance of anti-production such as the despot: capitalist social-production is organized by the market and for nothing other than the continuing production of surplus-value for its own sake. So at the same time that it re-organizes social-production in a completely distinctive way, via axiomatization – rather than merely appropriating the surplus from existing systems of production as despotism had done – capital becomes, as it were, its own instance of anti-production: surplus-value becomes an end in itself.[22]

Capitalist axiomatization, then, represents the second great deterritorialization of codes and meaning by abstract value (despotic tribute having been the first). And this time, with the institution of fully commercial (rather than mere tribute) money and the market, abstract value prevails – in the form of true exchange-value: money and axiomatization now *replace* codes and meaning as the basis of social organization, rather than remaining contained and controlled by them, as was the case in despotism. "Unlike previous social machines," Deleuze and Guattari explain, "the capitalist machine is incapable of providing a code that will apply to the whole of the social field. By substituting money for the very notion of a code, it has created an axiomatic of abstract quantities..." (33/41).

Social valuation is now quantitative rather than qualitative: exchange-value simply disregards or over-rides the concrete differences between commodities, rather than reducing them in the name of similarity and identity, as codes strive to do. Capitalist axioms conjoin quantified resource-flows to extract a differential surplus from their conjunction: whatever local codes may temporarily spring up in the process will be merely incidental and strictly subordinate to capital's axiomatic self-expansion. And so the form of coding characteristic of capitalism involves a contradictory process of *de*coding and *re*coding, whereby extant codes of meaning and conduct are swept away by a wave of axiomatization which generates a temporary recod-ification of new meanings and practices, that are themselves swept away in turn by the next wave of axiomatization, and so on. It is important to note that recoding (despite its morphology) is quite unlike coding and over-coding, for capitalism provides no stable codes capable of governing the whole social field: like decoding, recoding is a mere concomitant of axiomatiz-ation, not the principal means of organizing social-production on the socius, as were coding and over-coding. This is one reason why Deleuze and Guattari distinguish capitalist surplus-value as a surplus-value of flows – it involves immanent flows of quantified factors of production and consumption conjoined by axioms rather than codes or over-codes.

The relations of anti-production and systems of inscription

Now that we have outlined the two basic types of the social organization of matter- and energy- flows – direct and indirect, symbolic and economic – we can examine the three modes of social-production/anti-production themselves in more detail. In all three, forces of anti-production institute regimes of debt and social obligation that are designed to prevent the direct appropriation and immediate consumption of the fruits of social-production, as I have already suggested – but the means instituted to do so vary considerably. At the same time, a system of social inscription executes the specific type of social repression that each mode imposes on desiring-production:

> social inscription...on the socius is in fact the agent of a secondary psychic repression, or repression "in the proper sense of the term," that is necessarily situated in relation to the desiring-inscription of the body without organs, and in relation to the primary repression that the latter already performs in the domain of desire – a relation that is essentially variable. There is always social repression, but the apparatus of repression varies...

> (184/217–18)

I will examine first the relations of anti-production and systems of inscription of savagery and despotism, then turn attention to capitalism and the way it finally manages to impose its Oedipal inscription on desire.

Savagery (1): the relations of anti-production

In savage society, the forces of anti-production operate by means of kinship relations. However, what we call "kinship relations" are, under savagery, co-extensive with the organization of the social field as a whole (166/196); the nuclear family, and the reproductive functions occurring within it, are not segregated from social relations at large, as they have been under capitalism. Marriage functions not merely as a pairing of two individuals, based on personal predilection and undertaken primarily for the purpose of bearing and raising children, but as a fully social event implicated in and governed by the entire social order, undertaken so as to consolidate and/or ameliorate the positions of entire families and lineages within the savage community. Two important implications follow from the non-segregation of savage reproduction from social-production at large.

For one thing, what we know as the "incest-taboo" functions in a very different – not to say opposed – fashion in savage society. Whereas we think of the incest "taboo" as an injunction *against* sexual relations among family members, it functions in savage society, on the contrary, as an incitement *in favor of* making connections in the social field. Indeed, to speak of the

69

incest "taboo" as a prohibition, a *pro*scription bearing on reproduction, is already in a sense to impose a modern Oedipal perspective on savage social organization. For the social imperative under savagery is on the contrary pre-eminently positive: a *pre*scription to form or strengthen family alliances, to share or distribute wealth, to knit social ties, by insisting that the young find their spouses exogamously, outside of their own family group or clan. By contrast, incest appears to us as a taboo – a "dirty little secret" (269/320) – because reproduction in the nuclear family has been segregated from other social relations in such a way that family members become the most conspicuous objects of desire. The Oedipus becomes a *complex* for us in a way it could not have been for societies with extended rather than nuclear institutions of reproduction, where so much positive incentive and social importance attach to marrying outside the family group.

This is not to say that there is no taboo against incest in savage society, but rather that the negative *pro*scription is merely the corollary of a detailed and all-important *pre*scription to share, distribute, knit social ties. In fact – and this is the second implication of the coincidence of relations of reproduction and relations of social-production/anti-production in savage society – the *exact same kind of imperative* governs production and reproduction alike. Everyone must share or distribute the fruits of their labor; or conversely, no one may appropriate for themselves what they have produced – hunted, gathered, reaped – but must rather relinquish it to the network of debt-obligations that constitutes the very structure of the relations of savage anti-production.[23] What we call the incest-taboo thus represents a sub-category of a larger class of taboo which constitutes the law of savage anti-production and organizes both social-production and reproduction: hunters are forbidden to consume their own kill just as parents are forbidden to procreate with their own children. That the taboo bearing on reproduction seems so much more important to us than the taboo bearing on production is due to a kind of optical illusion: from our perspective, the taboo on production is moot because with specialization and the extensive division of labor characteristic of capitalism people, inevitably produce for the market, and *cannot* directly consume what they produce. Under savagery, relations of anti-production must enforce what the market system under capitalism seems able to ensure effortlessly and as a matter of course: that there will be no direct appropriation of the fruits of labor.

The general law of savage social organization, then, is that all means of life – wombs and material goods alike – must circulate. The system of savage debt-obligations and expenditures is established precisely in order to prevent desire from gaining immediate access to its object, which is life and the means of life. It is because immediate access is to be prevented by a mode of repression which turns desire away from its immediate aims that Deleuze and Guattari characterize savage social organization as "perverse." The relation of desire to its primordial objects, the sources of life itself – to the earth (food, clothing, shelter, etc.) as well as the mother (breast, placenta, womb, etc.) – must be mediated by the laws of social organization.[24] The productive synthesis of connection which would make immediate (and multiple) connections with mother and earth gets interrupted by the disjunctive synthesis of recording, which establishes the network of relations of anti-production comprising the savage social order.[25] This is, of course, an *exclusive* use of the disjunctive synthesis, for savage social organization actively encourages some relations and discourages others.

The general syntax, so to speak, of savage social organization comprises marriage alliances and lineage filiations, the synchrony and diachrony of kinship, if you will. Unlike the nuclear family in modern society, where filiation relations involve usually only two (or at most three) lineage generations and alliance relations go no further than one layer of "in-laws," savage lineages are calculated many generations deep, and savage alliance relations extend throughout the social field. Indeed, under the pressure of complex alliance patterns, kinship relations combine with myth to extend savage lineages all the way back to the earth itself, while the matrix of alliances become co-extensive with social organization as a whole. Since debt and expenditure obligations under savagery remain finite, mobile, and reciprocal, they form neither a closed system of exchange nor a fixed hierarchy permanently elevating one clan or group above the others. Determinate patterns of circulation produce only differences in rank, which arise from the ebb and flow of debt obligations, and are hence always subject to change.

Savagery (2): territorial inscription

Savage social organization is actualized by a system of inscription that Deleuze and Guattari call a system of "cruelty" (184/218). The temptation of direct appropriation of the matter- and energy-flows of life is so great and so immediate, and the requirement of obedience to the social group so strong, that the laws of savage anti-production – exogamy; no immediate consumption – are branded directly into the flesh of the body. Invoking the Nietzsche of *The Genealogy of Morals*, Deleuze and Guattari suggest that an enormous amount of pain and cruelty are required to forge a collective memory powerful enough to overcome the appeal of unmediated life (144–5/169–70). The main threat to savage society arises not from incest, they insist, but from flows of matter or energy that might escape capture by the forces of anti-production that constitute savage social organization; rituals of cruelty and systems of inscription are instituted precisely to *code* all matter- and energy-flows so that they circulate throughout society and cannot escape its grasp. Savage coding is thus linked *both* to the system of debt-obligations and expenditures it enforces and makes possible *and* to a specific form of "writing" that creates and imposes a collective memory on the savage tribe.[26]

Savage writing as a mode of inscription is distinctive in that it is characteristically performed on the body (or the body of the earth). Equally important, such writing is independent of spoken language: the voice and graphics form two formally independent sub-systems of inscription; neither serves as signifier for the other. Finally, voice and graphics are nevertheless brought together to inscribe savage law in more or less public rituals where an authoritative gaze (of a shaman, a specific social group, or the community as a whole) confirms acceptance into the community based on the pain suffered in the process of inscription. The gaze functions crucially to overcome the formal independence and to sanction the "arbitrary" conjunction of the other two components of the ritual, which Deleuze and Guattari therefore characterize as a system of *connotation* (203/241).

Deleuze and Guattari describe one such ritual, in which the clan of a young woman and that of her husband mark her body with an excision that will confirm the legitimacy of their alliance and act as a sign of its fertility:

> The calabash of...excision is placed on the body of the young woman. Furnished by the husband's lineage, the calabash serves as a conductor for the voice of alliance; but the graphism must be traced by a member of the young woman's clan. The articulation of the two elements takes place on the body itself, and constitutes the sign [of fertility].
>
> (188–9/223)

Deleuze and Guattari go on to insist that such a sign "is not a resemblance or imitation, nor an effect of a signifier, but rather a position and a production of desire" (189/223): the sign operates less to convey a message – the woman does not learn the meaning of the ideograms during the initiation rite – than to assign reproductive organs a place and a (hopefully fruitful) function within the group. Everyone henceforth knows to whom this womb belongs – or rather, exactly what position it occupies in the network of alliances and filiations of the society, and to whom its fruits will be due, along which pathways of debt and expenditure they will have to circulate.

Several features of savage society are worth underscoring for the sake of comparison with despotism and capitalism. For one thing, savage debt is open-ended, composed of what Deleuze and Guattari call "mobile and finite blocks of debt" (190/225). While it is true that savage myth supplements the reckoning of lineages so as to ground them in the earth itself, the system of alliances that constitute the network of debt-obligations is subject to constant renegotiation, and thus never forms a closed system. "A kinship system is not a [fixed] structure but a practice, a praxis, a method, and even a strategy," Deleuze and Guattari conclude; "[it] only appears closed [to exchangist anthropologists] to the extent that it is severed from the political and economic references that keep it open" (147–8/173).

For another thing, the voice and graphics form two independent systems, which rituals bring together in an a-signifying way under the gaze of the group (or of such sub-groups as are permitted to witness this or that ritual). Crucially, savage writing does not represent speech. Moreover, rituals of cruelty assign social place and function to specific organs by marking bodies or body-parts; whole persons are not at issue. A fertility ritual assigns the womb, and the womb alone, to its place in the relations of anti-production; which foods the young woman may eat, what stories she may tell or to whom she may talk are determined by various other rituals bearing on different organs of the body. Savage organs belong to the group rather than to private egos or selves (which only emerge later). In this context, incest as we know it (or rather as we conceive of it, according to the modern "incest-taboo") is in an important sense simply not possible: the organs of reproduction (and production, too) are first and foremost assigned a place and function in the social order; they belong not to an individual but to the group.[27] One result, it is true, of such assignment – but not the one directly aimed at – is that sexual relations among immediate family members are discouraged. But the "taboo" forbidding sexual relations between whole persons within the immediate family is merely an after-effect – or better, an after-image – of the primary assignment of place and function to specific, collectively invested organs within the community.

Deleuze and Guattari therefore conclude that the Oedipus plays no role in organizing savage society: Oedipal incest is only a negative after-image of the law which does in fact organize savage society (while also determining the development of extended lineages): the law of exogamy and the system of marriage-alliances it fosters. Here again, the tripartite semiotic of the poststructuralist critique of representation is critical: it enables Deleuze and Guattari to distinguish between the alliance–debt system as the *repressing representation* of desire, on one hand, and the taboo against incest which is the *displaced represented* of desire, produced by the repressing representation itself, on the other. Equally important, it enables them to distinguish both elements of representation from the immediate object of desire, the *representative of desire*, which as I have said is life itself and the means of life. Desire does indeed get repressed under savagery, very severely repressed; however, it is not incest but the desire for life that gets repressed, by being inscribed in a determinate social system of representation:

As for Oedipus in general [under savagery], it is not the repressed – that is, the representative of desire, which is on this side of and completely ignorant of daddy–mommy. Nor is it the repressing representation, which is beyond, and which renders [whole] persons discernible only by subjecting them to the...rules of alliance. Incest is only the retroactive effect of the repressing representation *on* the repressed representative: the representation disfigures or displaces

73

this representative....[I]t projects onto the representative [the] categories that it has itself established and rendered discernible; it
applies to the representative [specific] terms that did not exist before
the alliances organized...a system in extension...the representation
reduces the representative to what is blocked in this system. Hence
Oedipus is indeed the limit, but the displaced limit that now passes
into the interior of the socius. Oedipus is the baited image with
which desire allows itself to be caught (That's what you wanted!
The decoded flows were incest!). Then a long story begins, the story
of Oedipalization.

(165–6/195; translation modified)

But the decoded flows were not incest: they were life itself. The primary
function of savage representation is to code the un-coded flows of life, to
institute through rituals of cruelty a system of alliances and filiations in
order to prevent the direct and hence anti-social appropriation of life. Far
from playing a determining role in this system of repression, the Oedipus
appears only as an after-image, an internalized limit. As such, it begins what
we can see retrospectively as a long yet halting migration to replace life and
become the very representative of desire, which it finally does only under
capitalism. But first we must examine the entirely different relations of anti-
production and system of inscription characteristic of despotism, to
understand what they in turn contribute to the long story of Oedipalization.

Despotism (1): the relations of anti-production

In despotic society, the forces of anti-production operate via undisguised
political domination. Despotism results from conquest and the formation of
empires, and its mode of anti-production involves superimposing the relations of conquerors to conquered over the existing social dynamics of the
latter: "the essential action of the [despotic] State...is the creation of a
second inscription by which the new full body [of the despot]...appropriates
all the forces and agents of production" (198/235). Remnants of the older,
non-power, social relations remain in force locally and co-exist, to a greater
or lesser extent, with the new power-relations of the empire, but they do so
only within its limits, and so it is on these power-relations that we will focus
here.[28] In brief, whereas savage anti-production ensured the sharing of fruits
of labor, imperial anti-production enforces the extraction of tribute from its
subject-peoples for the sake of glorious expenditure (*dépense*) on the part of
the despot.

The general law of despotic social organization is not the savage law that
anything of value must circulate in horizontal circuits of debt and obligation, but that everything is owed to the despot. The despot imposes this
infinite and unilateral debt by transforming the general syntax of the savage

communities beneath him, seizing its patchwork of alliances and lineages and re-aligning all of them on himself. The figure of the despot thus replaces the earth as the socius and original ground of all lineages, in direct filiation with what is characteristically a monotheistic deity, and supplements the networks of savage alliance with a new alliance from above that links him not with this or that specific family or clan, but with his subject-peoples as a whole, and as an un-differentiated mass. Rather than owe one another reciprocal and dischargeable debts, they now all owe the despot everything.[29] This includes their lives, for one thing, inasmuch as the power of the despot includes the power of life and death over his people: under despotism, "the debt becomes a *debt of existence*, a debt of the existence of the subjects themselves" (197/234). And it includes tribute, of course, which although paid in money, as we have said, remains a surplus-value of code in that it is extracted by seizing the existing circuits of debt and expenditure obligations and turning them all toward the coffers the despot. But the infinite debt therefore also includes wombs and the women who bear them (e.g. the ten virgins "owed" to the Minotaur annually), inasmuch as they circulate in the very same circuits of debt and expenditure as material goods do.

Since subject-peoples now owe their despot everything, he has thereby gained the right of access to all women indiscriminately, regardless of their former lineage or erstwhile alliance obligations. The despot is in principle everyone's father, but equally everyone's son, brother, spouse. Hence the figure of incest, which had appeared as a mere after-image of positive marriage-inducements under savagery, now becomes in a sense ubiquitous and inevitable, if only symbolically, with the new-alliance and direct-filiation relations of despotism. But such incest is the exclusive prerogative of the despot: the right to incest is a power that sets him completely apart from ordinary mortals. One result is that incest in this "royal" or despotic form is no longer the *displaced represented* of desire, but has become the *repressing representation* itself. Imperial relations of anti-production are based on caste distinctions that separate the despot and his court retainers or state bureaucrats from everyone else. Incest now appears taboo for ordinary people precisely because it is the prerogative of the despot:

> In the imperial formation, *incest has ceased being the displaced represented of desire to become the repressing representation itself....*
> [The] way the despot has of committing incest, and of making it possible, in no way involves removing the apparatus of social and psychic repression [*l'appareil répression-refoulement*]. On the contrary, the despot's intervention forms part of the apparatus…a new economy in the repressive-repressing apparatus [*l'appareil refoulant répressif*], a new mark, a new severity. It would be…too easy if it were enough to make incest possible in this sovereign fashion for the exercise of psychic repression and the service of social repression

> to come to an end. [But] royal barbarian incest is merely the means
> of overcoding the flows of desire, certainly not a means of liber-
> ating them.
>
> (201–2/238–9; translation modified)

Royal incest is still not yet the incest of everyman's psychoanalytic Oedipus
complex (though we are one step closer), for this form of incest exercises its
mode of repression not by universally forbidding it but by making it licit for
the despot alone within a system of rigid caste distinctions.

The position of the despot, then, is in a literal sense an enviable one. He
concentrates in his person the function of anti-productive expenditure for
the entire empire and all of its peoples, and exercises the right of eminent
domain over everything they produce and reproduce, as well as over the very
life and death of the people themselves. Inasmuch as absolutely everything is
owed to the despot, and all organs, persons, and products belong to him as
parts of his full body, his transcendent position is inherently *paranoid*:

> Royal incest is inseparable from the intense multiplication of organs
> and their inscription on the new full body. The apparatus of social
> repression–psychic repression [*l'appareil de répression-refoulement*] –
> i.e. the repressing representation – now finds itself defined in terms
> of a supreme danger that expresses the representative on which it
> bears: the danger that [even] a single organ might flow outside the
> despotic body, that it might break away or escape.
>
> (210–11/249)

Given the paranoia of the despot's position, the *repressed representative* of
desire under the imperial regime of infinite debt can be none other than
betrayal, disobedience, eventually resistance and rebellion, and the despot
musters all the powers of coercion and representation to pre-empt them
all.[30] Indeed, having lost their capacity for self-determination after conquest,
as their savage codes get over-coded by imperial representation and their
alliances and filiations appropriated by the state, subject-peoples have been
effectively pacified: the threat of death they now have reason to fear arises
not so much from natural circumstance or the threat of ostracism from the
group (as under savagery) as from the despot who wields the power of life
and death over them; death no longer appears as an accident or a simple fact
of life, but now has become a permanent menace from on high, inflicted by
force of arms and backed by the imperial state and its system of law.
Obedience to the transcendent law of the despot is enforced not through
branding the flesh but by the threat of death:

> There occurs a detachment and elevation of the death instinct,
> which ceases to be coded in the interplay of savage actions and

reactions...in order to become the somber agent of overcoding, the detached object that hovers over each subject.

(213/252)

Deleuze and Guattari therefore call the imperial system of inscription a system of *terror* (211–13/250–2).

Despotism (2): imperial inscription

What is distinctive about this system of inscription is that the independence of voice and graphics characteristic of savagery disappears: writing now aligns itself on the voice, but on a voice that is crucially absent (as Derrida has shown is true for all writing). The imperial domain is too large to be governed in person, so the state administers by written decree. The one sub-system of inscription has now become the signifier of the other: writing moves into a position of visible dominance in practice, yet becomes subordinate to the absent voice it merely represents. Deleuze and Guattari thus call imperial inscription a system of *subordination* (205–9/243–8), to distinguish it from savage connotation. Two important consequences follow from the subordination of writing to voice.

The role of the eye in appreciating inscription has diminished immeasurably: it no longer seals the voice–graphics relation, appreciates the pain and sanctions the effects of ritual inscription; it merely reads what has been written (often in the foreign language of the conquerors). Body representations, Deleuze and Guattari say, have become subordinate to verbal representations (215/255). Moreover, in order to make sense of these signifiers of a mysterious written voice that speaks from on high, state subjects must have recourse to interpretation. Writing no longer directly designates valued objects of desire (organs of production and reproduction) while allocating them within the savage community; writing now entails wanting to know what an absent Other wants. A second pacification of despotic subjects takes place, accompanying the ever-present threat of death: desire no longer desires objects, but desires another's desire; desire has become desire of the despot's desire. Desire no longer acts in relation to the objects of value designated by collective ritual, but merely reacts to the written law promulgated by the despot:

> The complex relationship of designation...elaborated in the system of primitive connotation, with its interplay of voice, graphism, and eye, here disappears in the new relationship of barbarian subordination. How could [such] designation subsist when the sign has ceased to be a position of desire in order to become this imperial sign, a universal castration that welds desire to the law?

(214/253)

Here is a second answer to the questions raised in Chapter 2 about the historical conditions underlying the Lacanian account of desire: desire as desire of the Other's desire is the form of desire characteristic of power societies, not the nature of desire itself. Desire takes a very different form in savage society, as we have seen – and may take yet other forms under capitalism, except to the extent that state domination continues to hold sway.

For even when the state evolves from imperial tyranny toward republican democracy, its subject citizens will have recourse to this same law in their attempts to protect themselves from despotic excesses and secure a counter-power of their own. Desire in despotism has become thoroughly reactive, in the Nietzschean sense of the term: under the regime of infinite debt, as Deleuze and Guattari put it, "the eternal *ressentiment* of the subjects answers to the eternal vengeance of the despots" (214–15/254). The system of state terror, with its elevation of death to a permanent threat and its subordination of desire to the despot's desire, thus sponsors a massive pacification and a becoming-reactive of subjectivity – from which capitalist subjects, too, have yet to escape, inasmuch as the state survives the transition from despotism to capitalism in altered form, as we shall see.

But despotism is still not yet the domain of the Oedipus complex, although several more of its pieces are now in place. True, death has become a permanent threat; desire has indeed been severed from its object (life and means of life) only to become reactive, desire of another's desire, and to favor verbal representations over body representations: caste-enforced castration (caste-tration) has succeeded in welding desire to the law. Incest has indeed captured desire, but in a system where royal incest as repressing representation prohibits common incest as its displaced represented, and where the repressed representative of desire now appears as revolt against and freedom from the despot.[31] Oedipal incest has still not yet become the representative of desire itself – which occurs only under capitalism. So we now turn to examine the conditions that lead the Oedipus to complete its migration from the mere displaced represented (under savagery) to the repressing representation (under despotism) to become the very representative of desire, in a system where it will come to occupy all three positions.

Capitalist relations of anti-production

In capitalist society, the forces of anti-production operate through the market; the relations of anti-production are economic rather than personal: "the alliances and filiations no longer pass through people but through money" (264/315). As in despotism, the debt remains infinite, so that filiation still predominates over alliance, but its ground, the socius, is no longer the figure of the despot: it is capital – specifically industrial capital. And inasmuch as full-fledged industrial capitalism is the sole system of social-production that always produces too much (in its own terms, at least, which take no account of glorious expenditure), the social function of the debt and of the state changes significantly as well. For the state does not disappear under capitalism, even though it no longer represents a transcendent unity imposed from above: instead, it "becomes immanent to the field of social forces, enters into their service, and serves as a regulator of the decoded and axiomatized flows" (252/300). And anti-production functions not as an external damper or limitation on consumption but as an internal stimulus to consumption in the attempt to avoid crises of over-production.

> The apparatus of anti-production [under capitalism] is no longer a transcendent instance that opposes production, limits it, or checks it; on the contrary, it insinuates itself everywhere in the productive machine and becomes firmly wedded to it in order to regulate its productivity and realize surplus-value....[C]apitalism's supreme goal...is to introduce lack where there is always too much, by effecting the absorption of overabundant resources.
>
> (235/280)

Capitalist anti-production thus culminates not in the transcendent glory of, say, the Palace at Versailles, but in the morbid greed of what Deleuze and Guattari refer to as the "politico-military–industrial complex" (235/279), among other things. For what the production and especially the realization of surplus-value require, given the inherent tendency of capitalism to over-produce on a continually larger scale, is a vast system of anti-production installed at the heart of production itself to keep its wheels turning by absorbing over-production.[32] Such was the intended effect, for example, of Keynesian economic policy and the New Deal, though it was really achieved only by the Second World War and the nuclear arms race; and such is the ongoing function, Deleuze and Guattari suggest, of "advertising, civil government [including] the State, its police, and its army, militarism, and imperialism" (235/279). It is only when people can be convinced that they are lacking something (anything ranging from "the latest" fashion trend to "national security") that they can be induced to consume and produce at the ever-increasing rate the capitalist economy requires. The debt owed to capital remains, like that of despotism, uni-directional and infinite, but the system of anti-production under capitalism has become immanent to the system of production, and has as its motive force only further production of surplus-value for its own sake. Consumption as the realization of surplus-value is not an end in itself but merely the means of securing liquid capital for reinvestment in the next cycle of social-production.

Capitalist inscription

Given this indifference towards ends, and the replacement of coding and over-coding by axiomatization and decoding/recoding, Deleuze and Guattari will call the capitalist system of inscription a system of *cynicism* – though it does contain an admixture of (mostly false) *piety* to the extent that people continue to pretend to believe (in "progress," "technology," "life-style choice," "the end of history," or whatever), when in fact "there is no longer any need for beliefs [and] language no longer signifies something that must be believed [but] indicates instead what is going to be done" (250/298; translation modified). Cynicism and piety express the two moments of the capitalist form of coding – decoding and recoding – which in turn correspond to the two moments comprising the basic rhythm of capitalist axiomatization: deterritorialization and reterritorialization.[33]

Deleuze and Guattari consider decoding to be the positive moment of axiomatization, as I have said, because it frees desire from the constraints and distortions of codification. For schizoanalysis, one corollary of the immense productivity of capitalism admired by Marx is the freedom it grants practices from becoming fixed in established codes (the moment of cynicism). But the emancipatory effects of decoding which stem from the economic component of capitalism are accompanied by opposing processes of recoding stemming from its power component, which tie freed libidinal energy back onto factitious codes (the moment of piety) so as to extract and realize privately appropriable surplus-value. This opposition between decoding and recoding derives not so much from the classic nineteenth-century contradiction between the outright owners of capital and the dispossessed, as from the tension between the generally socialized production of surplus-value, on the one hand, and its private ownership and management, on the other. On the one hand, capitalism devotes itself to production as an end in itself, to developing the productivity of socialized labor to the utmost: this is the moment of deterritorialization. Yet, on the other hand, due to private investment in the means of production, social labor and life are restricted to production and consumption that valorize only the already-existing capital-stock: this is the moment of reterritorialization.

In the third volume of *Capital*, Marx outlines these two moments of capital's on-going self-expansion.[34] In a first moment, a wave of new, more productive capital-stock transforms the existing apparatuses of production and consumption; this "continual revolution of the means of production" that for Marx characterizes capitalism deterritorializes existing labor and capital in order to devote them to new forms of production and consumption, and in the process spawns decoding throughout society. But, in a second moment, this progressive movement is abruptly stopped, and everything is reterritorialized: the evolving apparatuses of production and consumption alike are tied down to what is now obsolete capital-stock, solely in order to valorize it and realize profit on previous investment. A wave of deterritorialization liberates all kinds of creative energies (in consumption as well as in production) at the same time as it revolutionizes and socializes productive forces; but then reterritorialization supervenes, yoking the relations of production and consumption to the dead-weight of private surplus-appropriation.

Reterritorialization thus actualizes the power component of capitalism, the retrograde force that hinders development of new productive forces and, more importantly, prevents the expenditure of surplus for purposes other than reinvestment in further surplus-production, while deterritorialization as the economic component represents the "constant revolutionizing of the means of production" that generates change and frees the energies of production and consumption from their existing objects and limitations. Of course, these terms express an analytic distinction between two "moments" of a single process (the process of axiomatization) that practically speaking occur simultaneously. The distinction is nonetheless crucial inasmuch as it highlights the difference between power and economics as two conflicting "moments" or components of capitalism.[35]

The relation between decoding and recoding is similar, but in a sense reversed. Both of these "moments," too, stem from axiomatization: decoding represents the positive moment of the process whereby desiring-production is freed from fixed codes, and recoding serves to recapture desire in facti-tious codes in the service of reterritorialization and capital accumulation. But whereas reterritorialization predominates under capitalism – capitalism can indeed be defined in opposition to communism simply as the contain-ment and command of productive forces (themselves developed through deterritorialization) by private appropriation (enforced through reterritorial-ization)[36] – recoding fails in Deleuze and Guattari's view to contain decoding, and remains a much weaker force than reterritorialization. This is because capitalism, as I have said, is basically meaningless, and axiomatiza-tion continually unleashes more decoded flows than recoding can recontain. Recoding is, to be sure, a reactive force that works to recapture and hence repress free-form desire in fixed codes, but since the capitalist socius orga-nizes quantified rather than coded flows, sign-systems in all media play at best a secondary role.

The capitalist system of inscription therefore derives not from the inter-relation of writing and voice, as in savagery and despotism, but from the dynamics of axiomatization: from deterritorialization and reterritorializa-tion, decoding and recoding.[37] And at the same time as it consigns writing and voice to the subsidiary moment of recoding, the capitalist market performs a thoroughgoing demotion of the family, for capital itself now takes charge of the functions of both social-production and social reproduc-tion, which had been the business of families and/or directly political domination by the state. Under savagery, of course, family, kinship, and social relations directly coincided; but even under despotism, relations within each caste were largely family-determined – whether by the residues of local coding for the subject-peoples, or by dynasties and the inheritance of titles for the despot and his minions – while the relation between them was patently political. Under capitalism, however, the once-dominant state, as we saw, becomes merely "the regulator of decoded flows as such, insofar as they are caught up in the axiomatic of capital" (252/299):

> [The state] was first this abstract unity that integrated subaggregates functioning separately; it is now subordinated to a field of forces whose flows it coordinates and whose autonomous relations of [class rather than caste] domination and subordination it expresses. It is no longer content to overcode maintained and imbricated territorialities; it must constitute, invent codes for the decoded flows of money, commodities, and private property.[38]
>
> (221/261)

Now, basic social ties are knit not familially, interpersonally, or politically but by the market.[39] Social-production and reproduction take place via the flows of money and capital. And since these decoded and axiomatized flows are governed by a purely quantitative calculus, most social roles now derive from economic functions, instead of simply coinciding with them. The important apparent exception is the family, which now occupies a "private" sphere segregated from social-production and reproduction in the "public" or economic sphere, with results I will return to in a moment.

Economic relations become dominant and largely supplant the political relations of despotism, meanwhile, through the transformation of merchant capitalism into industrial capitalism. Trade, commercial money, and exchange-value were able to co-exist with the tribute form of money within despotism, although this latter remained predominant (by definition). Merchant capitalists made profits through exchange by buying cheap in one place and selling dear in another: their operation depended on and derived from the independence of localities and differences between their price-structures. Deleuze and Guattari consider this an alliance form of capital, since it operates laterally in an open-ended and comparatively unsystematic way.

The great transformation occurs, Deleuze and Guattari agree with Marx, when abstract labor takes on real, practical existence with the commodification of labor-power: in schizoanalytic terms, capital becomes filiative. Before that, the exchange-value of commercial money represents a "mere" abstraction projected by the exchange-relation itself, and its potential dynamism could be contained by over-coding. Once industrial capital and commodified labor-power emerge, exchange-relations cease being open-ended and haphazard; value circulates through its various moments – money, commodities, means of production, labor-power as a commodity – without leaving the sphere of social-production or ceasing to be value.[40] And at the same time that the open-endedness of merchant capital gets subsumed by this completely integrated circuit of value, labor-power produces a surplus-value from within it, from within what is now a self-contained fully economic system, and industrial capital becomes the new socius at its center:

> In brief, the capitalist machine begins when capital ceases to be a capital of alliance to become filiative capital. Capital becomes filiative when money begets money, or value a surplus-value....It is solely under these conditions that capital becomes the...new socius...that appropriates all the productive forces.
>
> (227/269–70; translation modified)

Filiative capital has in effect taken the despot's place as focus and basis of social investments, and however extensive the lateral exchange-relations of alliance (trade) become as the market continually expands, the infinite debt is still owed to capital as the apparent source and ground of extended filiations based on the anticipated production of ever-greater quantities of surplus-value. The infinite debt owed to owners for past investment in effect mirrors the infinite production to which labor-power will be devoted, now and in the future. This is the context in which anti-production ceases being an end in itself, becomes immanent to production, functions merely to absorb excess product and insert consumption into the cycles of ever-expanding surplus-production: this is the context, in a word, in which *asceticism* – infinite labor to pay the infinite debt (akin to Weber's Protestant work ethic) – becomes the rule of capitalist subjectivity.

Yet the capitalist socius *per se* has no means of directly inculcating such asceticism: its purely abstract quantitative calculus is incompatible with the formation of subjectivity, which involves qualities, meanings, beliefs. Under capitalism, as Deleuze and Guattari put it,

> [r]epresentation no longer relates to a distinct object, but to productive activity itself. The socius...has become directly economic as money-capital....What is inscribed...is no longer the producers or non-producers [as person-objects] but the forces and means of production as abstract quantities that become concrete in their becoming related or their conjunction...
>
> (263/313)

So capital delegates the formation of subjects to the family. For at the same time that the operations of social-production and social-reproduction (via commercial trade-alliances and financial debt-filiations) are completely taken over by capital as the new socius, human reproduction alone is for the first time completely segregated from social-production/reproduction; human reproduction, that is to say, is henceforth privatized in the nuclear family.

The effects of such segregation are decisive. For one thing, with social reproduction governed by the market and divorced from human reproduction, the "incest-taboo" becomes for the first time purely negative: the imperative no longer has anything to do with knitting basic social ties or justifying and expressing glorious expenditure: it merely prohibits biological incest. In this respect, the nuclear incest-taboo adds an internalized – psychological – form of pacification to the political pacifications of despotism. But this capitalist form of pacification may be even more virulent, because desire gets caught from the very start in a grotesque double-bind: the isolation of the nuclear family from society at large segregates desire from all possible objects *except* the very ones that are prohibited, namely family members. Desire is forbidden access to precisely those objects that are, under the circumstances, the most desirable. The nuclear family thus provides a perfect training-ground for the ascetic subjectivity fostered and required by capitalist anti-production. What is more, the restricted and restrictive relations within the family do not just produce a generalized asceticism: *they reproduce in microcosm precisely the basic relations of capitalism itself*. For just as capital separates the worker from the means of life and defers gratification until after work, after pay-day, and after retirement, the castrating father separates the child from the nurturing mother and defers gratification until maturity and the founding of a new family:

> [When] the alliances and filiations no longer pass through people but through money...the family becomes a microcosm, suited to expressing what it no longer dominates [i.e. social reproduction].... [I]nstead of constituting and developing the dominant factors of social reproduction [as in savagery], [the family] is content to apply and envelop these factors in its own mode of reproduction. Father, mother, and child thus become the simulacrum of the images of capital ("'Mister Capital, Madame Earth,' and their child the Worker"), with the result that these images are no longer recognized at all in the desire that is determined to invest only their simulacrum. The familial determinations become the application of the social axiomatic. The family becomes the subaggregate to which the whole of the social field is applied.
>
> (264–5/315)

If social roles under capitalism are already images of economic functions, as we have said, family roles are merely "images of [these] images, derivatives of derivatives" (264/315). Capitalist subjects are trained in asceticism by an institution that is isolated from social repression, yet exactly reproduces capitalist social structure and dynamics in their most abstract terms. What is more, the capitalist family also reproduces the basic elements of social-repression from the other social formations: separation from the means of life, incarnated in the forbidden mother, and obedience to despotic law, incarnated in the forbidding father. The Oedipus *as complex* has arrived.

84

With the axiomatization of social-production and reproduction by capital and the ensuing segregation of human reproduction in the nuclear family, then, the Oedipus complex completely saturates the tripartite representation of the incest-taboo. Not only is incest the repressing representation and the displaced represented, as it was in despotism and savagery: it has become the very *representative* of desire, inasmuch as desire now as never before lives the threat of incest daily in the libidinally charged confines of the nuclear family.[41] As repressive as the other modes of libidinal production were, at least the representative of desire in those regimes had a different aim: direct appropriation of means of life under savagery; freedom through revolt against political domination under despotism. Of course, desire still takes these (and other) forms under capitalism – we still want to secure the means of life, and would still like to end political domination – but now the material institution of the nuclear family supplements the defiles of representation with an "objective" form in which to entrap desiring-production: the Oedipus complex.

If this last pacification of desire is indeed the most virulent and sinister of all, as I have suggested, it is because in one sense desire now no longer knows what it wants: material circumstances and repressing representations combine to offer desire the very familial objects that they simultaneously forbid: "Oedipus is the baited image with which desire allows itself to be caught" (166/195). What is more, the death instinct which first arose under despotism becomes even more pervasive under capitalism: instead of hovering over everyone as a distant threat from the despot, death now becomes immanent to everyday existence, which harbors the omnipresent threat of having insufficient money to secure food or shelter – the omnipresent threat, that is, of losing one's job, and so losing market access to the means of life. This market-based form of the death instinct, like the other elements of capitalist asceticism, is reflected and reinforced by the dynamics of the nuclear family, with parental love functioning as money: since children are effectively isolated from other sources of nourishment and protection, if they forfeit parental love, if they break the "law of the father" and lose access to the mother, they will perish.[42] Under both sets of conditions, the death instinct compels desire to become increasingly pacified and reactive: desire of another's desire – but now the boss's or the father's rather than the despot's.

In another and more important sense, however, desire always desires what it desires (partial-object relations), even when it does not know what it desires, or believes otherwise – as when, under determinate conditions, the institutionalized representative of desire is incest with whole-object persons:

> [Even] when the requisite conditions [for the Oedipus complex] are
> realized in capitalist society, it should not be thought on that account
> that Oedipus ceases to be what it is, the simple displaced represented

> that comes to usurp the place of the representative of desire, snaring
> the unconscious in the trap of its paralogisms, crushing the whole
> of desiring-production, replacing it with a system of beliefs.
> Oedipus is never a cause: it depends on a previous social investment
> of a certain type...
>
> (178/210–11)

The disparity between desiring-production and its institutional representation under capitalism is all the greater in that, while the family operates on persons, capitalist social-production operates by decoding and axiomatic conjunctions: it is not because of who they are as persons that some are destined to be the wage-slaves of others, but merely inasmuch as they are owners of some or none of the means of production, owners of capital or only of labor-power. With decoding operating at full-throttle in society at large, as we shall see in the next chapter, desire is freed from codification and depersonalized; the family, by contrast, is a major locus (though not the only one[43]) of recoding and the personification or "impersonation" of desire.

It is crucial to recall in this connection that although the nuclear family is segregated from society at large under capitalism, it is by no means autonomous or independent of it. On the contrary, the family is delegated its specific roles – recoding, formation of ascetic subjects, the pacification and impersonation of desire – by the mode of social-production. Deleuze and Guattari therefore insist that the Oedipus complex is not itself a cause, but a relay, entirely dependent on the mode of social investment of desire:

> It will be objected that such a principle [the primacy of social
> investment] is perhaps valid for the adult, but surely not for the
> child. But in effect, Oedipus begins in the mind of the father. And
> [even this] beginning is not absolute: it is only constituted starting
> from investments of the social historical field that are effected by
> the father....The fact that the father is first in relation to the child
> can only be understood analytically in terms of another primacy,
> that of social investments and counterinvestments in relation to
> familial investments.
>
> (178–9/211)

The Oedipus complex derives from the social formation, then, and gets delegated by it to the nuclear family as its agent for the formation of ascetic subjectivity. As noted in Chapter 2, without this crucially socio-historical perspective on the Oedipus and its program of pacification, any social repression becomes merely a "sublimation" of inevitable psychic repression, and "all resignations are justified in advance" (74/88).

The primacy of social investments of desire in relation to familial investments also explains why Deleuze and Guattari insist that psychoanalysis did not invent the Oedipus complex, that on the contrary "the subjects of psychoanalysis arrive already Oedipalized...[and] all [that psychoanalysis does] is reinforce the movement, add a last burst of energy to the displacement of the entire unconscious" (121/144). In this light, one of Freud's most dramatic discoveries turns out to be among his most pernicious: "the transference." For the Oedipus complex now appears as an internalized–psychologized version of subjection to despotic law and state domination: the castrating law of the father represents an internalized displacement of what I called the "caste-trating" law of the despot, carried out in circumstances of widespread decoding where political dominion no longer operates as directly in society at large. For subjects are now efficiently if abstractly disciplined, starting from birth, by the law of the father and that of the market: abnegate, identify, defer, and work – or perish. Yet the family is never completely segregated from decoding in society at large, and especially as the insularity of the family increasingly succumbs to the forces of socialization and axiomatization through mass education, the mass media, etc., familial recoding and paternal authority weaken in their turn – and so psychoanalysis steps into the breach to shore up the Oedipus complex, instead of accepting (much less promoting) the decoding of desire. The law of the father was already a displaced substitute for the law of the despot as *his* power diminished in the face of axiomatic decoding; now, via the transference, the psychoanalyst will in turn substitute for the father as the latter's influence also wanes in the face of decoding. In effect, when the familial subjection of desire falters, psychoanalysis steps in to offer a partially axiomatized variant, aligned on and supportive of the familial Oedipus, but now based on exchanging correct beliefs and behavior for money rather than for parental love. To the (very considerable) extent, then, that its therapeutic practice and its theory are organized around transference, the nuclear family, and the Oedipus complex, Deleuze and Guattari insist that psychoanalysis must be understood as a strictly capitalist institution. For the Oedipus as complex is the specific representation that capitalist social-production offers desiring-production as the representative, the repressing representation, and the displaced represented of desire, precisely in order to repress it – and psychoanalysis serves mostly to reproduce this structure and reinforce its effects.

Schizoanalysis and Freud

By showing how psychoanalysis participates in and contributes to capitalist subjectification in these ways, schizoanalysis is able to bring psychoanalysis to the point of autocritique. But this does not constitute a wholesale condemnation of psychoanalysis; far from it. Many of the concepts, and some of the procedures, of psychoanalysis remain crucial to schizoanalysis – libido, free-association, and primal repression, most notably – even while others are rejected as misguided or self-defeating – most importantly sublimation, transference, the death instinct, and the Oedipus complex understood as universal rather than as the capitalist repressing representation of desire.

Freud's greatest discovery, as I have said, was of libido as the abstract, subjective essence of desire, free from specific objects pre-determined to be "desirable," and instead bestowing libidinal value upon its objects through fluid investments of desire: free-form libido makes legitimate use of the unconscious syntheses. But Freud then betrays his own greatest discovery, and assigns desire universal predetermined objects and aims: sex with the mother and identification with the father – the Oedipus complex. And, in doing so, Freud merely reproduces the institutional structure of capitalist reproduction: in the nuclear family desire has, in fact, been segregated from society at large, in an illegitimate use of the conjunctive synthesis, so that libido is tied down or recoded onto family members as the principal objects of desire. No such segregation occurs, by contrast, in savage society, where desire invests the entire social field by way of the patchwork of alliances and filiations, and in the form of partial-object organs that circulate throughout that patchwork in place of whole-object persons; nor does it occur under despotism, which ultimately focuses desire on the distant figure of the despot himself, but without sealing off human reproduction from the rest of society altogether, as in the nuclear family.

The idea of free-association, similarly, implies legitimate use of the connective and disjunctive syntheses. In (truly free) free-association, open-ended chains of multiple signs would arise and could intersect at random with other chains, without being reducible to a single meaning or representative. Yet, under capitalism, almost all signs except those of parental figures are decoded by the market, so that illegitimate segregation combined with such decoding serves to reduce the multiplicity of signs to just a few, which resonate out of all proportion to their real importance within the confines of the Oedipal triangle. Freud reinforces this extraction and elevation of a few privileged signs from an initial multiplicity in what was referred to in Chapter 2 as the second and fourth paralogisms of psychoanalysis, the paralogisms of application and extrapolation, by constantly forcing the Oedipal interpretation on the polyvocal semiotics of free-association. Furthermore, such restriction induces an illegitimately exclusive use of the disjunctive synthesis, whereby desire must choose between two objects of attraction and identification: the same- or opposite-sex parent; the prohibitor or the prohibited. This structure of invidious distinction, where one belongs either to the elite or to the masses, first arose under despotism, but does not yet completely envelop and determine desire there, inasmuch as the local imbrication of human with social reproduction is left more or less intact. It is only when, under capitalism, this large-scale either/or structure migrates into the heart of the nuclear family that the illegitimately exclusive disjunction effectively captures desire in a double-bind, as the authority of the despot devolves onto the forbidding father, and the mother becomes the forbidden fruit of gratification. In this circumstance, Freud sees no alternatives for desire other than fixation within the original Oedipus complex or its "resolution" in the formation of another Oedipus complex in the next generation: this is the third paralogism of psychoanalysis, the paralogism of the double-bind.

The concept of primal repression (*refoulement originaire*), finally, helps explain how it is that desire both differs from pure instinctual determination and becomes susceptible to capture by representation in the first place. But the crucial ambivalence of primal repression – which enables us to critically evaluate the effects of specific representations on desiring-production and justifies efforts to intervene in the process of representation – is betrayed when primal repression is confused with one socio-historically specific repressing representation of desire, *viz.* the Oedipus complex, which is then used to justify such repression as universal and therefore inevitable. Here Freud mobilizes the fifth paralogism of psychoanalysis, the paralogism of the afterward, which in effect reverses the direction of determination: social repression, in Freud's view, becomes a mere "sublimation" of original Oedipal repression.

All the paralogisms are in a sense underwritten and made possible by the first one, the paralogism of displacement, whereby psychoanalysis mistakes the true nature of desire for what the repressing representations of all three modes of social-production forbid, that is, mistakes desire for the displaced represented of repressing representation, confuses the nature of libido with the Oedipus complex. In short, where psychoanalysis has gone most wrong, it has fallen prey to the ruse of representation, albeit an "objective" representation reflecting the segregative structure of capitalist society, since the Oedipus is indeed the way desire is actually lived at the heart of the nuclear family.

Schizoanalysis and Lacan

Yet here the figure of Lacan stands as an important exception: no one has done so much within psychoanalysis to call into question the strategies and effects of representation in Freud and in psychoanalytic discourse in general. For, according to Lacan, the Oedipus complex in conventional psychoanalytic discourse is an Imaginary representation of psychic structure and dynamics – to which he counterposes a Symbolic or structural version that takes into account the semiosis (or at least the linguistics) of desire. But the question remains, just how critical will Lacan's Symbolic version of the Oedipus prove? Deleuze and Guattari invoke the story of the Resistance fighters sabotaging a bridge who place explosive charges so precisely under the pylons that the whole thing blows sky-high, only to fall right back into place exactly as they found it. Schizoanalysis, by contrast, will want to ensure that the autocritique of the Oedipus is *irreversible*.

As we saw in Chapter 2, Lacan's structural Oedipus complex translates concrete parental roles into more abstract linguistic existential functions. For better or for worse, Lacan's Oedipus will function regardless of whether or not the particular personalities of the parents or the culture of child-rearing conform to Freud's rather Victorian vision of family life. Separation from the mother now means losing touch with the substance of the body or "being" as one enters the realm of language and meaning in the Symbolic Order; the castrating prohibition against incest (le "non/nom du père") becomes homonymous with the father's name, which as signifier designates both the exclusive phallic right to the mother and the position the male child will come to occupy; and so on. Yet the genealogy of modes of social-production presented in Chapter Three of *Anti-Oedipus* reveals that the elements and functions of this structural-linguistic version of the Oedipus have socio-historical origins, too. The mother's body as lost realm of substance and being derives from the lost territory of savagery, where partial-object coding remained immanent to social relations of production and reproduction, not governed from above by a detached transcendent term. The castrating law of the father, in the same vein, derives from the caste-trating law of the despot, and the role of the paternal metaphor or signifier corresponds to despotic over-coding. Desire under castration is mediated desire of the transcendent Other's desire; the infinite debt owed this intimate transcendent Other sponsors the metonymy of desire as search for substitute partial-objects through a process of recoding sanctioned by the name-of-the-father. A modern intimate form of despotic decree, the unconscious has come to resemble an oracular text without a voice, the meaning of which many a psychoanalyst, functioning as a kind of priest or elite functionary, will help decipher.

Yet for the radical therapeutic practice of Lacan himself, the unconscious text has no meaning, the place of the Other is really empty, and the thera-pist's role is to make sure it stays empty. This role of the therapist as "sujet-supposé-savoir" – the subject who is supposed by the analysand to know, but in fact does not – exploits an ambiguity in the functions of the Other within the Symbolic and Imaginary registers, an ambiguity that is crucial to the practice of psychoanalytic therapy as Lacan construed it. From the standpoint of the Symbolic register, the Other designates only a place; but in the transference that place is occupied by the person of the analyst, who becomes an Imaginary Other to the analysand. The aim of the Lacanian analyst in this position is not to reinforce but to dismantle the transference – to dissolve, from the *place* of the Other, the *figure* of the Imaginary Other projected onto the analyst by the patient, and thereby restore the subject to its relations in the Symbolic Order.

From the perspective of schizoanalysis, then, Lacan must be (mis?)understood as shouldering the mantle of the despot in the transference – invoking the Law, desire as desire of desire, castration, lack, loss of being, and so on – solely in order to expose its functioning and get rid of it, in order to blow it up and blow it away. And if the place of the Other in the Symbolic register is construed as empty, that is because capitalist axiomatization and decoding continually undermine all social meaning and authority (including the father's); under these circumstances, any attempt to re-establish meaning and authority through recoding and the transference appears as an Imaginary illusion, perhaps even a paranoid delusion.

The main thrust of Deleuze and Guattari's genealogical critique of the Oedipus, then, is to break out of the stifling confines of the nuclear family, and restore the analysis of desire to its full socio-historical context, "to discover beneath the familial reduction the nature of the social investments of the unconscious" (271/323). Once the Oedipus complex is understood as the application of essentially capitalist social investments to the intimate sphere of the family,[44] the tasks of schizoanalysis are to examine how axiomatization, decoding, and recoding themselves inform desire, and to explore the conditions under which the untrammeled desire of schizophrenia could be marshaled to counteract and dispel the forces of paranoia in society at large. With the genealogical critique of Oedipus now behind us, we can turn to these more general tasks.

4

BEYOND CRITIQUE
Schizoanalysis and universal history

For schizoanalysis, the mode of functioning of the psyche is crucially ambiva-lent: the process of recording on the body-without-organs frees desire from instinctual or habitual determination (by breaking organ–machine connec-tions) yet, at the same, it time makes desire susceptible to capture in repressive social representations (by inscribing desire in the terms offered or imposed by society). The body-without-organs acts as a kind of "pivot" or "frontier" (281/334), as Deleuze and Guattari put it, between desiring-production and its social inscription. What is distinctive and significant about the capitalist mode of social inscription in comparison with the other modes is that its functioning, too, is ambivalent or contradictory: capitalist axiomatization entails both deterritorialization and reterritorialization; and capitalist repre-sentation raises the ambivalence of the psychic recording process to a maximum, by sponsoring both decoding and recoding. Capitalism thus inaugurates the *possibility* of universal history: it frees labor and libido from illusory objective determinations, revealing the abstract subjective essence of production in both fields, desiring-production and social-production. But, at the same time, capitalism prevents and defers the *realization* of universal history by re-subjecting free productive energy to the alienations of private property and the privatized family, to capital and the Oedipus.[1]

Hence one of the paradoxes of capitalism: the *identity in nature* of desiring-production and social-production is revealed in the same mode of production where the *difference in regime* between the two is the greatest. The other modes of production assigned desire and labor to pre-established objects of investment (the earth, the despot); and since human reproduction was still integral to social reproduction, the family remained a fully social institution. The abstract subjective essence of labor and desire remained hidden due to their objectification in and by codes, yet they both belonged to the same overall regime of coding. Capitalism has no such overarching code: axiomatization operates instead on decoded flows of abstract labor sundered from all pre-established objective determinations, at the same time as human reproduction is segregated from social reproduction in the nuclear family, which renders desire abstract as well. Such segregation has

92

the additional effect of making the one appear completely separate from the other: desire and labor henceforth apparently belong to entirely different regimes of production: desiring-production and social-production.[2]

The two modes of investment: paranoia and schizophrenia

Unlike the other modes of production, then, which did their utmost to code or over-code desire and channel its investment into pre-assigned objects, the capitalist socius supports *two different kinds* of investment: one corresponding to the liberation of abstract subjective desire and labor by deterritorialization and decoding, the other corresponding to the resuscitation of temporary artificial territories and codes through reterritorialization and recoding. This difference is so fundamental that Deleuze and Guattari present it as a basic thesis of schizoanalysis, in fact the last of the four theses they present in Chapter Four of *Anti-Oedipus*[3]: there are under capitalism "two poles of social libidinal investment," *paranoia* and *schizophrenia*. Schizophrenia – arising from the movement of deterritorialization and decoding – designates free-form desire in the psyche and the potential for universal history under capitalism, while paranoia – corresponding to reterritorialization and artificial recoding – designates the obstacles to realizing this potential that are imposed by private capital accumulation.[4] Crucially, these are no longer psychiatric terms, for reasons expressed in the first and third theses of schizoanalysis: that every psychic investment is simultaneously a social investment (despite the apparent segregation of familial desire from society at large); and, furthermore, that the social aspect of the investment is always determinant (despite the familial terms in which psychic investments most often get expressed, given the "representative" role of the nuclear family under capitalism).[5] Each pole of social libidinal investment can therefore be analyzed in terms of its characteristic mode of psychic functioning as well as its social function.

Within the psyche, schizophrenia and paranoia designate two forms of libidinal investment or processing on the body-without-organs: one that is polyvocal, free from coding, over-coding and recoding, the other coded and therefore univocal. In both cases, desire registers in the psyche, but in one case the moment of registration is simply an occasion to set desire in motion again to make other connections on other trajectories, whereas in the other it serves to fix desire in determinate (usually socially sanctioned) representations that henceforth govern which connections will and will not be made. In both types of investment, the same syntheses are at work, Deleuze and Guattari insist, but what they call the *molecular* form of schizophrenic investment makes legitimate use of the syntheses, while the *molar* form of paranoid investment makes illegitimate use of them.[6]

The distinction between molar and molecular investments does not correspond at all to the division between individual and society (280/332–3):

molar and molecular instances co-exist on the body-without-organs, and indeed they are almost always very closely imbricated. Deleuze and Guattari go so far as to say that "molecular desiring-machines are in themselves the investment of large molar machines or of the configurations that desiring-machines *form according to the laws of large numbers*" (287/342). The ambivalence of the recording-process on the body-without-organs here takes on added significance.

In one sense, molar investments are simply ones that happen to corre-spond to prevailing social norms and to thereby reinforce what Deleuze and Guattari refer to as "gregarity" or "herd instinct" (287/341–2 and *passim*), whereas molecular investments depart from and thereby can subvert those norms. And if molecular investments do (by definition) subvert norms, it is ultimately because they differ *in form* from molar investments (365–6/438–9): molecular recording disjunctions are inclusive rather than exclusive, their machinic connections multiple and partial rather than global and specific, their subject-conjunctions nomadic rather than sedimented – and so desire remains multi-variable and polyvocal instead of succumbing to univocity and belief.

In another sense, however, molar investments do not express merely statistical regularities or aggregates: herd instinct or forms of social gregarity exert strong selective pressure on molecularity to limit its multiplicity and shape it to prevailing forms of sovereignty (full sovereignty under savagery and despotism; ambivalent "neo-sovereignty" in the case of capitalism). Molecular desire is what is given; "'culture' as a selective process of marking or inscription invents the large numbers in whose favor it is exerted" (343/410): molar forms operate by capturing molecular desire in representa-tions whose force results from the process of selection itself. The ambivalence of primal repression (*refoulement originaire*) succumbs to over-determination by social repression (*répression*) operating within the psyche on the body-without-organs.[7]

If we turn now to the social function of the two kinds of investment, molar-paranoid and molecular-schizophrenic, it should be clear that capi-talism stands out from the other two social forms, which were single-minded about blocking the free-form desire of schizophrenia by capturing and over-determining desiring-production in codes and over-codes enforced by cruelty and terror. Capitalism, by contrast, is ambivalent: it borrows para-noia from despotism, as we saw, in conjunction with its drive to reterritorialize and recode; yet at the same time it promotes schizophrenia in its inevitable propensity to deterritorialize and decode. And it earns its inaugural position in universal history on the side of decoding and schizophrenia, as I have said.

Deleuze and Guattari's notion of universal history is quite specific, based in part on comments Marx makes in *Grundrisse* (1939), where he insists that "world history has not always existed; history as world history [is] a result" (109). Like schizophrenia and the body-without-organs, according to Deleuze and Guattari, universal (or what Marx here calls "world") history arises only at the end of history – as capitalism reveals the common essence of desire and labor, and then becomes capable of autocritique regarding the ways it nevertheless continues to re-alienate that essence (through capital and the Oedipus).[8] Yet that common essence is itself not fixed or determinate: desiring-production free from alienating forms of social-production (schizophrenia free from paranoia; market dynamics free from power) is the motor of permanent revolution, a movement of perpetual transformation and differentiation.

Schizoanalytic universal history thus involves difference rather than identity, singularity and escape rather than unity and reconciliation.[9] And the subject of this history is not a class destined to put an end to all classes, and thereby found a harmonious society no longer riven by class conflict and exploitation, but the molecular unconscious of the human animal as biological life-form. In this respect, Deleuze and Guattari's materialism appears closer to that of Nietzsche or Spinoza than that of Marx (except perhaps in the latter's notion of "species-being"). For the unity of humanity and nature is based on understanding history as the cyclical reproduction of life itself, with the unconscious ultimately taking the form of the genetic code.[10] This molecular unconscious as life-force represents the principle of difference and freedom – or of freedom as difference – beneath the conditions of identity required by consciousness and representation. And capitalism, for the first time in history (in a universal history it itself produces for the first time), frees the molecular unconscious from objective alienation in codes and over-codes, even though it strives at the same time to re-contain it, as we have seen, through recoding and reterritorialization. Bringing capitalism – the third mode of social-production in the semantic *combinatoire* presented in Figure 3.1 – to the point of autocritique thus projects a fourth mode, here designated as "permanent revolution." Whereas capitalist ambivalence combines the freedom of economics with the tyranny of power, permanent revolution eliminates power and paranoia in order to give free play to schizophrenia and enable molecular investments of desire to prevail over molar ones.[11]

Power and paranoia arise with despotism when the patchwork of mobile debts and alliances characteristic of savagery get over-coded by the infinite debt owed to the despot, thereby elevating filiation-relations centered on the despot to precedence over the alliances. The threat of death from ostracism in continuously negotiable social relations succumbs to a non-negotiable relation of allegiance and subjugation where the threat of death by execution at the command of the despot hovers over subjects as a form of permanent terror. Yet death and the expense of life still have a visible social presence and a prime social function, not only in public executions but in the despot's own glorious display of extravagance – a waste of life resources that sets him apart, as supreme agent of anti-production, from the common people and subjects them to his rule. Under capitalism, in turn, the infinite debt continues to subject the multitudes to social obligation, but death and expenditure lose all social primacy: social organization is devoted to production for production's sake (for the sake of surplus-value) rather than expenditure; anti-production, as we saw, gets subordinated to production, and serves merely to prevent recurrent crises of over-production from interfering with capital accumulation and self-expansion.

It is under these conditions, Deleuze and Guattari argue, that death becomes a silent yet omni-present "instinct," as Freud calls it: omni-present inasmuch as anti-production suffuses production throughout the production–realization–accumulation cycles of capitalist expansion; silent inasmuch as anti-production thereby becomes completely subordinate to production. Once the infinite debt and anti-production get subsumed by capitalist production, death is no longer a finite part of life, a moment of every becoming, but a permanent threat.[12] Moreover, although in principle production produces means of life, capitalist production produces not principally means of life but further means of production: production serves the avoidance of death rather than life itself; nothing can die, everything must be capitalized on and expanded. Death and expenditure now play secondary social roles, at best: mostly in the rampant militarism that absorbs surplus-production to forestall crises of over-production and keep the wheels of industry turning, when that surplus is not simply devoted to re-investment in further means of production. Along with consumption and reproduction, then, death too becomes privatized under capitalism: it no longer has social significance in a society devoted so completely to production. "Life" – a perverted version of life shorn of its intrinsic relation to death[13] – is so over-emphasized that pure expenditure gets repressed and death becomes "instinctual."

The logic of the fourth term in Deleuze and Guattari's semantic *combinatoire*, permanent revolution, therefore suggests not only a new combination of economics with non-power but a return to alliance-based social relations in order to re-establish the mobility and social value of death and expenditure – which occur sporadically both in savagery and on the body-without-organs, but which are monopolized and then repressed by despotism and capitalism, respectively. The return to alliance-based social relations in a post-capitalist market society would restore mobility to death and expenditure by making debts finite again, by making them dischargeable and renewable (unlike the permanent debt owed to capital). Market alliances free from the infinite filiation-debt to capital (in the form of negotiated contracts and the like) would be based not on socially imposed forms of obligation or necessity but on choice, opportunity, and freedom. Anti-production on the fourth socius would thus operate much as it does on the body-without-organs, enabling social connections and investments to be made, un-made, and re-made in accordance with the movements of molecular desiring-production itself. And this would require canceling the debt to capital, and hence making molar reterritorialization and recoding subordinate to molecular deterritorialization and decoding, rather than the other way round.[14]

Therapeutic transformation

The critical or destructive task of schizoanalysis thus extends beyond the critique of the Oedipus, on which we concentrated in Chapter 3 and from which *Anti-Oedipus* gets its name, to target reterritorialization, recoding, and paranoia wherever they operate – bringing not just psychoanalysis to the point of autocritique but contemporary society as a whole, in several of its major determinations: Oedipal, ascetic, capitalist.[15] Indeed, in line with the third thesis of schizoanalysis (which assigns social investments causal priority over familial ones, [356/427]), Deleuze and Guattari insist that Oedipus is not itself determinant of anything, but is rather "born of an application or reduction [of social dynamics] to personalized images, which presupposes an investment of a paranoiac type....Oedipus is a dependency of the paranoiac territoriality" (278/331). Reterritorialization fosters paranoid investments in society at large that restrict access to socially produced flows – you must refrain from appropriating collectively what you have collectively produced: thou shalt not murder the boss; thou shalt not expropriate the expropriators and re-appropriate the fruits of production. This type of investment is then applied to the nuclear family, which reproduces its substance and dynamics in a more abstract and even more restrictive form: thou shalt not murder thy father; thou shalt not re-appropriate thy mother (or siblings) – and no one else matters.

In this connection, Freud's critique of Jungian interpretation of symbolism in myth and tragedy is right, but only half-right. "Rather than referring symbolic representations to determinate objectities [*objectités*] and objective social conditions," Deleuze and Guattari explain, Freud "refers them to the subjective and universal essence of desire as libido" (301/359). But he then proceeds to draw on myth and tragedy to impose his own universal interpretation (the Oedipus complex) on the workings of the unconscious:

> [T]he ambiguity of psychoanalysis in relation to myth and tragedy has the following explanation: psychoanalysis undoes them as objective representations, and discovers in them the figures of a subjective universal libido; but it reanimates them, and promotes them as subjective representations that extend the mythic and tragic contents to infinity....[I]n fact, dream and fantasy are to myth and tragedy as private property is to public property.[16]
>
> (304/362)

Thus even though the Oedipal form of paranoia derives from capitalist society, it does not do so directly – as it would if it found adequate expression in myth or tragedy: for psychoanalysis and for modern man, the Oedipus appears only as fantasy, albeit a putatively universal one.[17] "Psychoanalysis and the Oedipus complex gather up all...that has ever been believed by humanity, but only in order to raise it to the condition of a *denial* that preserves belief without believing in it" (304/362–3): a last privatized piety for an otherwise thoroughly cynical age. Psychoanalysis appears in this light as a subjective recoding of an otherwise decoded and outmoded objective schema of representation – but is no less virulent a repressing-representation for it. And Lacanian structural psychoanalysis only abstracts and attenuates the same belief-without-believing, as the family as social institution succumbs to decoding and deterritorialization; for even reducing or expanding the Oedipus from family romance to linguistic metaphor, Deleuze and Guattari insist, "affords us no means for escaping familialism [but instead] attributes a universal metaphoric value to the family at the very moment it has lost its objective literal values" (307/366). Whether in the form of myth, tragedy, dream, or metaphor, the Oedipus is a representation and a belief (however attenuated) that functions to capture and distort free-form desire in fixed images.

But the unconscious itself is not concerned with belief, according to schizoanalysis. It does not want or believe anything: all the unconscious does is make and break connections, appropriate and redirect flows. The unconscious is available only through conscious representations, yet we can conclude nothing concrete about the unconscious from such representations: as Deleuze and Guattari insist, we cannot deduce the nature of desire from the content of conscious prohibitions against it or representations of it. We are still pious or paranoid as long as we believe in any univocal meaning or representation, given that contemporary society, based as it is on axiomatization, operates beneath or beyond the threshold of representation altogether. You can believe you are guilty of wanting to kill your father and sleep with your mother, you can believe in the Oedipus; but you can also believe you are guilty of not working hard enough, owing too much, or over-indulging yourself; you can believe in the superiority of your religion, nation, or sports-team – and all these beliefs are paranoid molar investments which contravene the molecular investments of desiring-production. Psychoanalysis did not invent Oedipus, as we have seen, but in circumstances where widespread decoding undermines its means of reproduction in the nuclear family, psychoanalysis nevertheless "fills the following function: causing beliefs to survive even after repudiation; causing those who no longer believe in anything to continue believing" (314/374), even if only in their private or metaphorical Oedipus. The critical task of schizoanalysis, then, is to destroy the power of representation in all its many forms, including the Oedipus complex, the ego, religious and ethnic fanaticisms, patriotism, the debt to capital, and so on; the aim is to expunge belief from the unconscious altogether, to undo molar recoding as much as possible.[18]

And what is possible in this respect, as has already been suggested, is undoing recoding to the point of subordinating molar to molecular forms of investment. Total escape from molar formations is neither necessary nor possible (since humans are by nature social animals); what is desirable, as suggested in Chapter 1, is that molar investments express to the greatest extent possible the movement and dynamics of the molecular unconscious: schizoanalysis is critical in a Kantian sense, as I have said, but brings this critique to bear on society rather than epistemology. Thus the corresponding positive task of schizoanalysis is to locate desiring-machines beneath or behind the systems of representation that capture and crush them, and to restore them to their proper molecular functioning:

> The task of schizoanalysis is that of learning what a subject's desiring-machines are, how they work, with what syntheses, what bursts of energy, what constituent misfires, with what flows, what chains, and what becomings in each case. [And] this positive task cannot be separated from indispensable destructions, the destruction of the molar aggregates, the structures and representations that prevent the machine from functioning.[19]

(338/404)

The therapeutic side of schizoanalysis, then, combines positive and negative tasks, corresponding roughly to the moments of decoding and recoding in society at large: on the one hand, to subvert molar investments and free subjects from the paranoid and/or pious beliefs that keep them subjugated to the alienations of private property imposed by capitalist recoding; on the other hand, to discover and develop molecular investments that express and promote the free-form schizophrenia of desiring-production released by market decoding. The aim, in short, is to release molecular desire from the constraints of molar representation.

Revolutionary transformation

The therapeutic component of the schizoanalytic endeavor is, however, strictly speaking inseparable from its revolutionary component, for (to recall the first and third theses of schizoanalysis) every psychic investment – whether paranoid or schizophrenic – is simultaneously a social investment, and indeed is first and foremost a social investment, even though it may be consciously perceived or expressed in personal or familial terms. Releasing schizophrenic desire from molar capture requires defeating the forces of paranoia throughout society, from the intimate confines of the nuclear family right up to and including the debt to capital: it requires full-scale social revolution.

Deleuze and Guattari's notion of revolution is, perhaps surprisingly, derived at least as much from Marx's materialist counter-parts, Nietzsche and Freud, as from Marx himself. For the basic premisses of schizoanalytic revolution are these: that the revolution will be anti-ascetic just as much as anti-capitalist; and that it will spring from the force of desire, not just a sense of historical duty or class interest.[20] Desire is part of the infrastructure (345/413; 348/416), and

> sexuality is everywhere: the way a bureaucrat fondles his records, a judge administers justice, a businessman causes money to circulate; the way the bourgeoisie fucks the proletariat....And there is no need to resort to metaphors, any more than for the libido to go by way of metamorphoses [i.e. sublimation]. Hitler got the fascists sexually aroused. Flags, nations, armies, banks get a lot of people aroused.
>
> (293/348)

Given the ubiquity and indeed the primacy of desire for schizoanalysis, then, "a revolutionary machine is nothing if it does not acquire at least as much force as these coercive machines [nations, armies, banks] have for producing breaks and mobilizing flows" (293/348). As much from its source in free-form schizophrenic desire as from its target in the asceticism of capitalist neo-sovereignty, revolution according to schizoanalysis necessarily entails the mobilization of libidinal energies.

This does not mean, Deleuze and Guattari are quick to point out, that they consider schizophrenics to be revolutionaries: they do not romantically idealize schizophrenia and madness as being revolutionary in themselves. For schizoanalysis carefully distinguishes between "the" schizophrenic as a clinical entity and schizophrenia as process:

> There is a whole world of difference between the schizo and the revolutionary: the difference between the one who escapes, and the one who knows how to make what he is escaping escape.... The schizo is not the revolutionary, but the schizophrenic process – in terms of which the schizo [as clinical entity] is merely the interruption, or the continuation in the void – is the potential for revolution.[21]
>
> (341/408)

It is not the entity but the process that has revolutionary potential – the process of molecular investment of the socius whereby free-form desire can subvert the molar formations of power and paranoia.

Moreover, Deleuze and Guattari are careful to insist that schizophrenia is the *potential* for revolution, not the revolution itself – and this for two reasons. For one thing, everything depends on the context and outcome of the schizophrenic process: on whether it gets interrupted or can proceed only in isolation ("in the void"), on the one hand, or can actively subvert molar formations and intersect with other decoded flows of social substance, on the other. Equally important, it is in the very nature of schizophrenia as free-form desire that it cannot be assigned any goal or end: schizophrenic desire in its opposition to paranoia is polyvocal, multiple, inclusive, non-specific, and nomadic, as we have seen. In line with Nietzsche's analysis of will-to-power, goals and ends for schizoanalysis always *issue from* desire, anyway, even though they appear (in consciousness) to guide it: submitting desire to pre-conceived goals would make it reactive rather than productive and creative. It is for this reason that Deleuze and Guattari insist that "schizoanalysis *as such* has strictly no political program to propose" and that it "does not raise the problem of the nature of the socius to come out of the revolution" (380/456).[22] For to do so would be to assign a goal to schizophrenia as process, and thereby subject the polyvocal molecularity of desire to univocal molar representation. The critical question they do raise bears on the "forms of conciliation" that any socius enables between desiring-production and social-production, with the general stipulation understood that permanent revolution would require the subordination of social-production and its form of sovereignty to molecular forms of desiring- production.[23]

The subordination of the specifically capitalist form of neo-sovereignty and asceticism to desiring-production would, as I have suggested, entail (among other things) cancellation of the infinite debt to capital and a return to alliance-based rather than filiation-based social relations. Yet the major difficulty in realizing the revolutionary potential of schizophrenia-as-process stems from the very primacy of desire that makes schizophrenic desiring-production so crucial. For what attracts desire, what ultimately governs libidinal investment, is the "degree of development of the forces or energies" that a given form of sovereignty is able to organize (345/413).[24] And capitalism, among all such social forms, has developed and organized the energies and forces under its command to a historically unprecedented degree. Indeed, it was able to effect its own revolution, according to schizoanalysis, precisely and only because it could develop the "productive forces" (forces of all kinds: economic, political, cultural, etc.) to a greater degree than could feudalism or absolute monarchy. The question thus becomes: under what circumstances and in what form can we imagine a socius emerging that would be more potent, in terms of the development of productive forces and energies, than capital? Deleuze and Guattari are not inclined to speculate on this question. But they do give the prospective socius to follow capitalism the epithet "new earth" (131/155; 299/356; 318–19/380–1; 321–2/384) – which suggests that a revolution may occur only after capitalist super-exploitation of resources has so severely impaired or even reversed its ability to continue developing productive forces and energies that some other mode of social relation to the earth shows visible signs of doing better. I will return to this prospect below, in connection with environmentalism.

In the meantime, the primacy of desire has important consequences for revolutionary strategy, as suggested by the second thesis of schizoanalysis, which distinguishes "the unconscious libidinal investment of group or desire [from] the preconscious investment of class or interest" (343/411).[25] For schizoanalysis assigns absolute priority to the former: although both levels or moments of libidinal investment are recognized as important, the unconscious investments of desire are fundamental; "[i]nterest always comes after" (346/415). This follows from Nietzsche's insight that consciousness and its preconceptions are epiphenomena of larger unconscious forces, which he refers to as will-to-power.[26] As Deleuze and Guattari put it:

> the unconscious libidinal investment is what causes us to look for our interest in one place rather than another, to fix our aims on a given path, convinced that this is where our chances lie – since love impels us in this direction. The manifest syntheses are merely the preconscious indicators of a degree of development; the apparent interests and aims are merely the preconscious exponents of a social full body.
>
> (345/413; translation modified)

What desire invests first of all and most fundamentally is not this or that object, nor this or that objective, but a *degree of development of force*, even though such force is usually most easily and widely accessible through the power-structure or form of sovereignty that developed and organizes it. (Capitalism is unusual if not unique in that its market mechanisms sometimes grant access to the productive forces of capital outside the established structures of power – even though the exceptions are usually short-lived and get quickly axiomatized in the service of further capital accumulation and expansion.[27]) The degree of development of force is primary: for what that force is used – its goals, aims, and the corresponding interests of those invested in it – is strictly secondary; it will always get rationalized *ex post facto*. Desire and interests co-exist, and interests have an undeniable role to play: for it is "under the cover of aims and interests" that desire invests the social full body. Nonetheless, "[t]he fact remains that there exists a disinterested love of the social machine, of the form of power, and of the degree of development in and for themselves" (346/414), and it is this love or desire, however absurd or "irrational," that is determinant.[28]

The second thesis of schizoanalysis thus helps explain Deleuze and Guattari's answer to Reich's question regarding fascism: the masses were not tricked; they desired fascism – and fascism wouldn't have succeeded for a moment without that desire, without that libidinal investment. But such investment is not for Deleuze and Guattari a matter of "ideology," of interests misunderstood or led astray. It is rather a matter of desire, and of how and where desire could invest a greater degree of force and power – even from a distance or indeed against one's "interests": "the most disadvantaged, the most excluded members of society invest with passion the system that oppresses them, and they always *find* an interest in it, since it is there that they search for and measure it" (346/415; translation modified). One can posit revolution as the "objective" interest of the masses or the working-class and be perfectly correct; but the real question, the one that schizoanalysis raises with such acuity and tenacity, is under what circumstances that interest corresponds to or becomes their desire, and conversely how that desire can so easily get captured and taken in quite the opposite direction.[29]

Desire and interest always co-exist, then, but do not necessarily coincide. Not only do "objective" and "subjective" interest often diverge but, more significantly for schizoanalysis, unconscious desire and preconscious interest may not coincide. Preconscious investments may be revolutionary in content or objective, yet molar and repressive in form: "a group may be revolutionary from the standpoint of class interest and its preconscious investments, but not be so – and even remain fascist and police-like – from the standpoint of its libidinal investments" (348/417). Deleuze and Guattari thus distinguish not only between the two moments or levels of investment – unconscious and preconscious – but also between two corresponding kinds of revolutionary break or rupture. A preconscious revolutionary break operates in the service of and with a view toward a new socius, with new aims and interests, new forms of codification or axiomatization, new forms of power. An unconscious revolutionary break, by contrast, operates in the promotion of molecular desire, subordinating molar forms to the subversive free-play of desiring-production. For revolution to occur, the two kinds of break must coincide: no revolution is conceivable without the definition of aims and the mobilization of interests; but no revolution ever takes place without the investment of desire.[30] Yet which of the two kinds of break ultimately prevails is crucial, for it determines whether the revolution will "go bad" and erect a new and equally or even more repressive power-structure (as usually happens, since the degree of development of force has increased in the process), or on the contrary will finally succeed in raising molecular desiring-production to predominance over herd instinct and molar gregarity, thereby realizing permanent revolution.

Revolution is prosecuted, then, by different kinds of group-formation, which Deleuze and Guattari call "subject-groups" and "subjugated groups" (drawing explicitly on Sartre's analyses in *The Critique of Dialectical Reason*[31]). And this distinction leads back to the difference posited in the fourth thesis of schizoanalysis, between the two poles of libidinal investment: the schizophrenic and the paranoiac. Subject-groups are characterized by unconscious investments of schizophrenic form, while subjugated groups operate according to preconscious investments of paranoid form:

The two poles are defined, *the one* by the enslavement of production and the desiring-machines to the gregarious aggregates that they constitute on a large scale under a given form of sovereignty; *the other* by the inverse subordination [of molar aggregates to desiring-production] and the overthrow of power. *The one* by these molar structured aggregates that crush singularities, select them, and regularize those they retain in codes or axiomatics; *the other* by the molecular multiplicities of singularities that on the contrary treat the large aggregates as so many useful materials for their own elaborations. *The one* by the lines of integration and territorialization that arrest the flows, constrict them, turn them back, break them according to the limits interior to the system...*the other* by lines of escape that follow the decoded and deterritorialized flows, inventing their own nonfigurative breaks or schizzes that produce new flows, always breaching the coded wall or the territorialized limit that separates them from desiring-production.

(366–7/439–40)

Generally speaking, subject-groups pursue unconscious revolutionary breaks, while subjugated groups only manage preconscious ones – even when they are successfully bringing about a revolution. But a given group can also alter its mode of functioning, passing from subject-group to subjugated group, and vice versa.[32] For this reason, Deleuze and Guattari insist on distinguishing between the form of libidinal investment – paranoid or schizophrenic – and the actual historical impact of group activity: a group can indeed produce revolution even as its form of investment oscillates between schizophrenic and paranoid or evolves (as often happens) from the one to the other.[33] However, only a consistently schizophrenic investment will sustain an unconscious revolutionary break, multiply its resonances and effects, and produce permanent revolution.

We are now in a position to understand the range of what can happen when subject-groups are able to follow through and make use of the decoded and deterritorialized flows unleashed by capitalism: Perhaps the worst-case result is that they escape from dominant aggregations and pass unproductively "into the void," so that the schizophrenic investments involved have no social repercussions whatsoever. Better, they can "make what they are escaping escape" by subverting the dominant aggregations and their representations while in the process of escaping them, if only temporarily. For, in most cases, such subversion gets absorbed – axiomatized and reterritorialized – by the existing system, which simply adds one more axiom to its structure of domination-appropriation (e.g. trade-unionism, Fordism, or the French Communist Party as ways of absorbing various workers' movements). Better still, subject-groups may amplify subversive decoding and deterritorialization to the point of inducing or abetting a preconscious revolutionary

104

break in the service of a new system of codification/axiomatization – in which case, however, the subject-groups eventually reassume subjugated-group form in the erection of a new power-structure, or are ruthlessly eliminated when other, already-subjugated groups seize power. Finally, it may be possible that subject-groups would produce an unconscious revolutionary break and then be able to sustain it: permanent revolution; the realization of universal history.

In all but the first (unproductive) and last (heretofore unrealized) instances, capitalist reterritorialization prevails and the subject-group either dissolves or is transformed into a subjugated group: it comes to see itself as permanent rather than transient (represses its own death); it assigns itself long-term aims and goals and thus defers fulfillment of desire, instead of acting immediately in situation (it begins operating strategically instead of tactically[34]); it forms exclusive and exclusionary inside/outside boundaries (via separation-segregation) rather than continually making, breaking, and re-making new connections with society at large; it develops an internal hierarchy and promotes identification with an authority-figure, along with disdain for outsiders.

It should come as no surprise that subjugated groups operating this way in the service of capitalist axiomatization and reterritorialization constitute a favored stomping-ground for successfully Oedipalized subjects from the nuclear family, for virtually the *same* pattern of repressionn–deferral–separation–abnegation–identification obtains in both cases. What appeared earlier as an abstract homology between the dynamic structures of capital and the nuclear family (" 'Mister Capital, Madame Earth,' and their child the Worker" [264/315]) is in fact a pattern materially produced and reproduced throughout capitalist society by subjugated groups in institutions of all kinds: political parties, scout troops, bureaucracies, sports-teams, armies, and last but certainly not least – the nuclear family.[35] Rare, indeed, is the group in contemporary society that is not a subjugated one – and lasts long enough to be noticed. The paranoia of the Oedipus complex, it was said, is an idea that begins not in the child, but in the mind of the father; yet that beginning itself "is not absolute: it is only constituted starting from investments of the social historical field which are made by the father" (178/211).[36] Those investments are not made solely in capital as socius, as the abstract form and dynamic governing society at large, but also in myriad intermediary institutions operating as subjugated groups.[37] The father conveys or relays a paranoid investment in the Oedipus complex not just because he lives under capitalism and reproduces within a capitalist institution (the nuclear family) but because he is invested and participates in subjugated groups throughout his everyday existence, and so reproduces their dynamics at home as well as nearly everywhere else.[38]

Happily, as ubiquitous as they are, subjugated groups under capitalism only ever have one leg to stand on: decoding and deterritorialization are constantly pulling the rug out from under any permanent formation (including those of capital itself). And that is where the chances for revolution lie, according to Deleuze and Guattari: on the side of the molecular and the schizophrenic. Schizo-revolutionary strategy thus seeks to reinforce and magnify the subversive thrust of capitalist decoding and deterritorialization; to provoke the transmutation or schism of subjugated groups into subject-groups; to "assemble its desiring-machines and its subject-groups in the enclaves or at the periphery" (277/329) so as to attain critical mass and overthrow power: to free desiring-production from molar social-production and ultimately subordinate the latter to the former.

Intersections

Hence the importance of provoking intersections among multiple lines of escape, so that they become "collective, positive, and creative" (367/440), rather than turn silently in the void or simply fizzle out. Deleuze and Guattari consider modernist art, science, and mathematics (each of which they cite consistently throughout the book) as strong vectors of decoding–deterritorialization which nevertheless remain axiomatized, and ask under what conditions their vectors of escape might intersect with and reinforce others in contemporary society, including psychiatry, workers' movements, and so forth.[39] In this final section of the book, I want to consider possible intersections of schizoanalysis with Marxism, environmentalism, and feminism. The point will not be to subsume these other movements under the banner of schizoanalysis but to suggest where and how schizo-revolutionary strategy may overlap with and/or depart from their concerns and objectives.

Marxism

Schizoanalysis draws selectively on Marx for its critique of Freud and oedipal psychoanalysis, as I have said. But at the same time it draws selectively on Nietzsche in ways that interfere with certain aspects of conventional Marxism. We have already encountered some of these ways: for one thing, Deleuze and Guattari consider ideology to be of far less importance than desire. People are not ideologically tricked into acting against their best interests: their *desire* is attracted by an organization of force that enslaves them; "[i]nterest always comes after" (346/415). The masses were not duped by fascism, Deleuze and Guattari agree with Reich: they actively desired it. In the same vein, schizoanalysis insists that revolutions are made by desire, not just duty or interest, and that the desire for revolution proceeds from a fundamentally visceral attraction to regimes assuring a greater degree of development of force.[40] As in the case of Nietzsche's will-to-power, conscious rationalizations in defense of a given social arrangement as well as formulations of the aims of a revolutionary undertaking arise *ex post facto*; the irresistible attraction of a greater degree of force is always primary. Finally, the subject of revolution and of universal history, according to Deleuze and Guattari, is neither a class nor humanity "as a whole" but the genetic unconscious as biological life-force. For schizoanalysis, "species-being" refers to the reproduction of the molecular unconscious and to the development of life-force, not to any specific qualities inherent in humankind.[41]

Schizoanalysis, we have also seen, distinguishes subject-groups from subjugated groups, and generally speaking favors the former over the latter. Political parties, organized as they are into subjugated groups, tend to repress free-form desire far more than do subject-groups, such as those involved in art movements, or even mathematical or scientific innovation (to the extent and so long as any of these groups are able to forestall axiomatization by capital). Deleuze and Guattari do recognize the importance and even the necessity of vanguard political organization: a revolutionary class, they say,

> can constitute itself only by a counterinvestment that creates its own interest in terms of new social aims, new organs and means, a new possible state of social syntheses. Whence the necessity for the other class to be represented by a party apparatus that assigns these aims and means, and effects a revolutionary break in the preconscious domain – the Leninist break, for example.
>
> (344/411–12)

Yet this very necessity merely displaces the distinction between subject-group and subjugated group. For "the class from the standpoint of praxis is infinitely less numerous or less extensive than the class taken in its theoretical determination" (344/412): even if the party apparatus operates internally as a subject-group, it functions as a vanguard by representing the masses' interests to the masses themselves, and by formulating their aims and means, thereby constituting or confirming the masses as a subjugated-group. And even when a revolutionary break has been effected, it is usually only a matter of time before the revolutionary subject-group mutates into or is supplanted by a subjugated group, with the erection of a new power-structure and matrix of repressive social representation.

The party and its vanguard are not, however, the only models available of revolutionary political organization. Movements and programs such as *autonomia* in Italy, *autogestion* in France, and direct or economic democracy and women's movements in the United States all present or propose less centralized and hierarchical forms of political organization – forms that would presumably or by definition remain closer to the mode of functioning of subject-groups. Antonio Negri has provided probably the most extensive Marxist analysis and rationale for this kind of group activity, and while we cannot reproduce his arguments in detail here, what can be said is this: drawing on the distinction Marx made between an earlier stage of merely "formal subsumption" of labor by capital and a more fully developed stage of capitalism where "real subsumption" prevails, Negri argues that with real subsumption, not just labor but all social activity falls under the sway of capital.[42] The production of value, the reproduction of labor, and the production-reproduction of suitable capitalist relations of production permeate all aspects of society. The real subsumption of labor and society by capital corresponds, in other words, to what Deleuze and Guattari call the saturation of society by capitalist axioms and the state's becoming immanent to capitalist production-reproduction. Society has become a "social factory," as Negri puts it, and surplus-value can now be extracted everywhere (in consumption and reproduction as well as production), not just in factories themselves.

Under the conditions of real subsumption, Negri insists, the fight against capital takes place throughout society: industrial labor at the factory no longer (for better or for worse) has a privileged position. So rather than a centralized hierarchy directing actions from above (as in most trade-union organizations and party formations), the *autonomia* movement recommended immediate re-appropriation of the fruits of socialized labor whenever and wherever possible, throughout society. These spontaneous or at most loosely coordinated actions closely approximate the mode of activity of Deleuze and Guattari's subject-groups, operating in "guerrilla" fashion against the power of capital. It should perhaps be acknowledged that the *autonomia* movement never attained the critical mass necessary to actually transform capitalism into something else. But such is the predicament of any and every subject-group in a capital-saturated society: how to move from effective but localized subversion to out-and-out revolution, without reproducing power relations and/or getting subsumed under a new capitalist axiom.

Hakim Bey sidesteps this dilemma in proposing what he calls "Temporary Autonomous Zones": eschewing any revolutionary ambitions (and working outside the Marxist tradition), he nonetheless recognizes the potential for freedom or autonomy inherent in contemporary society. Like Deleuze and Guattari (though without acknowledging the role of market decoding), he recommends that groups assemble to realize that potential for as long as possible, but without aspiring to permanence, thereby avoiding degeneration into subjugated groups, but also sacrificing any likelihood of full-scale transformation. The conundrum shared by all these thinkers seems to be this: utopian vision for now seems to outstrip real possibilities; the exceptional political forms that correspond best to the nature of desiring-production seem to have little chance of transforming social conditions permanently so that they could become the rule rather than the exception. No wonder Deleuze and Guattari insist that schizoanalysis has no political program!

The other major area of intersection between schizoanalysis and Marxism involves the notions of universal history and historical materialism. Deleuze and Guattari draw directly on Marx, as we saw, to criticize and historicize

Freud: he discovered libido as the abstract subjective essence of desire, but then re-alienated desire in the Oedipus complex, just as Smith and Ricardo discovered the abstract subjective essence of value, and then re-alienated it in private property. Both discoveries became possible when capitalism had made all of production abstract, through decoding and deterritorialization, even while it sundered the one from the other by segregating human repro-duction (libidinal economy) from social-production (political economy). Capitalism makes universal history possible, yet at the same time hinders its realization by recoding and reterritorializing for the sake of private surplus accumulation. Realizing universal history, according to Deleuze and Guattari, requires bringing both psychoanalysis and bourgeois political economy to the point of auto-critique, targeting asceticism and axiomatization in theory, and eliminating them in practice.

This view of universal history, as was suggested earlier, is quite unlike Hegelian philosophy of history, the simple "materialist" inversion of which constitutes some Marxist philosophies of history. For schizoanalysis, universal history is the history of chance and contingency, the elevation of difference and multiplicity to predominance over unity and reconciliation. Following Althusser, Deleuze and Guattari refuse all Hegelianism in their selective appropriations from Marx, and draw instead on the materialism of Spinoza. What is distinctive about Spinoza's view, in this connection, is that it is reso-lutely non-teleological – and thus offers a sharp contrast and alternative to Hegel's view. Given the contribution of Spinoza to Deleuze and Guattari's materialism, it is worth considering in some detail the alternative to Hegel that he represents.

The charges against Hegelian philosophy of history, especially within Marxism, are well-known: idealism, in that its starting-point, ending-point, and main actor are Spirit or Mind; transcendental subjectivism, in that this historical agent, Absolute Spirit, is a subject that transcends any and all concrete subjects and indeed history itself; teleologism, in that the end of history is guaranteed by the dialectical process of negation of the negation, so that even errors and mishaps eventually contribute to the realization of Absolute Spirit through history. And yet much of what passes as "Marxist" philosophy of history – including some (though not all) of Marx's own – merely translates or inverts Hegelian idealism into a "materialism" that nonetheless retains the transcendental subjectivism and the teleologism: classes act as transcendental subjects in the historical dialectic of class struggle, which will according to necessary laws produce a classless society with the collapse of capitalism at the end of history. This grand eschatolog-ical narrative, it should be noted, no longer inspires total confidence, even among Marxists. And it is in this connection that Spinoza appears as an alternative to Hegel and, by implication, to Hegelian Marxism.

To be true alternatives, however, Spinoza and Hegel must have something in common: in fact, the basic principle they share is that thought and matter are *ultimately* identical. But the forms of this "ultimate identity" are very different. In place of Hegel's idealism (which submits matter to thought via the "negation of the negation"), Spinoza offers a position that is certainly anti-idealist, if not actually materialist. Rather than elevate thought over matter (or matter over thought, as in a simple "materialist" inversion of idealism), Spinoza considers thought and matter to be absolutely *co-equal*: thought and extension are different but not opposed ("non opposita sed diversa") modes of substance. And as modes of the same unique substance their identity is given – whereas for Hegel, the identity of Spirit and matter is achieved only at the end of history. Even more important, thought for Spinoza is a property of substance, not of a subject; in place of Hegel's transcendental subjectivism, Spinoza offers a kind of immanent objectivism, for which no negativity and no contradiction are possible or necessary. (The success of Cartesian geometry and Spinoza's own practice as an optician and lens-grinder no doubt contributed considerably to his conviction that the universe is knowable in its own terms, that it has mathematical "thought" as one of its innate properties.) The Spinozan universe, then, is objectively knowable; knowability is one of its inherent features.

But whether such objective knowability is ever subjectively realized in human thinking is a very different question for Spinoza: it depends on humans overcoming through critical reflection the subjective limitations of what he calls "imagination" (and Althusser, "ideology"), thereby enabling knowledge to emerge that more closely approximates the "objective" thought inherent in substance itself. The development of adequate ideas does not follow automatically from the march of Spirit and the ruse of reason, but depends on humans' ability to distance themselves from the distortions of subject-centered thinking. This ability varies (socially, politically, historically), and is in no way guaranteed to increase through history. So in place of Hegel's teleologism Spinoza offers only the *possibility* that humans will forgo the illusions of subject-centered imagination and develop more adequate knowledge.

Finally – and this is where Spinoza's materialism comes into play – the prime measure of such adequacy is not some ultimate reconciliation of Spirit and matter, but rather the degree to which human capacities (*potentia*) are realized and increased. Humankind is a determinate mode of objective substance just like everything else in nature, and as such (according to the principle Spinoza calls *conatus* – "striving" – which Deleuze likens to Nietzsche's will-to-power[43]) it tends to develop its capacities to the utmost. What distinguishes humans is that, by acting in the mode of thought as well as of extension, they are able to understand, submit to, participate in, and thereby develop the forces of nature, of which they nonetheless always remain a part. Unlike imagination, adequate thinking furthers human–natural development rather than hindering it.

The view of universal history Deleuze and Guattari derive from the incorporation of Spinoza (along with Nietzsche, Marx, and Freud) into their version of "historical materialism" bears some resemblance to the Marxian view that posits a dialectic of forces and relations of production instead of class struggle as the "motor of history." This is perhaps the least Hegelian of Marx's several philosophies of history, inasmuch as it eschews the transcendental subjectivism and the teleologism of the class-struggle model.[44] For it is not a matter here of a contradiction between antithetical class-subjects necessarily leading to the synthesis of classless society, but of a tension between two ensembles – forces and relations of production – that not only are not subjectivities themselves but cut across class boundaries altogether.[45] Yet this Marxian model still contains residual elements of transcendental subjectivism and teleologism: a certain subjectivism inasmuch as the development of these human-centered productive forces, with something like "species-being" (homo faber) rather than classes as transcendental subject, is still considered the motor of history (though not necessarily its telos, which is rather the realization of human freedom presumed to depend on the development of productive forces[46]); and teleologism inasmuch as stagnant production relations, according to this model, necessarily come into conflict at some point with productive forces that nevertheless continue to develop, thereby eventually causing a revolutionary explosion which eliminates the old relations and replaces them with others better able to continue developing the productive forces. Schizoanalysis proposes to eliminate these residuals in two ways.

First of all, for Deleuze and Guattari the "productive forces" at issue in history are not exclusively or primarily those of humankind, but those of nature as a whole, of which humankind is of course an integral part, but only a part. Schizoanalysis thus offers a kind of anti-humanism (perhaps even more thoroughgoing than Althusser's own) that would impel Marxism to eschew "productivism" (i.e. the exclusive focus on production for production's sake) and consider humankind (as Marx himself sometimes does[47]) to be a part of nature rather than, in Hegelian fashion, its Master. It is in this vein that Deleuze and Guattari insist that "Nature = History = Industry" (25/32) and that the subject of history (of history as "natural history") is ultimately life, the reproduction of the molecular unconscious.[48] Second, and especially with "productive forces" understood to mean those of nature broadly construed (i.e. including but not limited to humankind), schizoanalytic materialism completely removes the inevitability of revolution and the progressivism of historical process itself. For there is no guarantee that human thought will continually or even consistently achieve the objectivity required to help rather than hinder the development of productive forces. There is no guarantee, in other words, that developing marketable productive forces will necessarily break the shackles of stagnant production relations: universal history is a history of contingency; and revolution occurs, as we have said, if and only if desire invests a new and different regime of social syntheses with a greater degree of development of productive force. In this respect, the schizoanalytic view of history is based more on Nietzsche and Spinoza than on (a still-too-Hegelian) Marx.

Environmentalism

Spinoza provides schizoanalysis with an alternative not just to Hegelian philosophy of history but to subject–object dualism in general. Spinoza was a contemporary and a critic of Descartes, and his view of the objective identity of thought and extension contrasts sharply with Descartes' view, which treats thought as a property of a doubting subject rather than of concrete objects. This critique of and "monist" alternative to Cartesian subject–object dualism represents an important contribution to contemporary environmentalism, since Spinoza insists on considering humankind a part of nature rather than its master.[49] Drawing in part on Spinoza, schizoanalysis considers the subject–object distinction to be secondary, as well: subjects and objects arise only in the third synthesis (the synthesis of conjunction), well after productive connections between humans and the environment have been made, their signs have been registered in the unconscious, and their important qualities (exclusive v. inclusive, multiple v. specific, segregative v. nomadic, etc.) thereby established.[50] Indeed, the ultimate identity of nature, history, and industry posited by Deleuze and Guattari already suggests fruitful intersections between schizoanalysis and environmentalism.

Yet the intersection of schizoanalysis with environmentalism is based at least as much on its appropriation of Bataille as on Spinoza. As we have said, Bataille takes as his point of departure the astro-nomical amount of heat- and light-energy our planet receives from the sun. A fundamental law thus governs what he calls the "biosphere": this energy must be expended. Various life-forms and various social forms have different ways of embodying, appropriating, organizing, concentrating, and expending their part of the excess energy-flows transiting the planet. Each life-form or social form expands to the extent its production–appropriation–consumption of resources makes possible within the limits set by the environment. Capitalism defies the law of "natural history" in that its form of social organization subordinates expenditure (anti-production) to surplus-production, as we have seen, and continually displaces any limits on further production by adding more and more axioms to its socius. Hence the importance for schizoanalysis of adding an emphasis on anti-production to the Marxist emphasis on production: only by targeting both the asceticism and the productivism that derive from the subordination of anti-production under capitalism, according to schizoanalysis, can there be hope for averting environmental catastrophe.

For the subordination of anti-production under capitalism has both psychological and socio-historical consequences. Psychologically, death becomes an "instinct," as we have seen: instead of being directly experienced in public expenditures of life and resources, it gets privatized and repressed. Directed inwards, the repressed death instinct returns as the neurotic guilt of the Oedipus complex and the asceticism required and fostered by capitalist surplus-production; directed outward, it returns as the drive for mastery and domination, visited upon other humans and the natural environment alike.[51] Socio-historically, the subordination of anti-production results in "productivism": capitalism not only develops its productive forces for the sake of surplus-production rather than expenditure, but counts as productive forces in the first place, only those it can register in its accounting system and thereby profit from, notably labor and technology; the "productive forces" of nature – resources such as clean air and water, fossil-fuel reserves, species diversity, and ecosystem integrity – are for the most part left out of the equation altogether. This restricted accounting system is important to Deleuze and Guattari's understanding of the dynamics of and limits to capitalist expansion, and therefore warrants closer examination. The issue here is whether limits to capitalist development, if indeed any exist, are primarily economic or environmental.

The capitalist system of commodity-production treats everything as if it were a commodity, even though much of what enters the system is not produced as commodities. This is notably true of human labor itself, which is inserted into production as a purchased commodity (labor-power) even though it is (re)produced outside the sphere of production: in the family (and perhaps the education system).[52] But it is even more clearly true of resources such as air and water. Even when states attempt to regulate their exploitation by assigning values to them (via taxation or fines, for instance), such valuations are not strictly speaking market valuations: they cannot be calculated in terms of cost of production, because such resources are not produced as commodities. Human and natural resources are therefore in an important sense *preconditions* of production which enter into the system of commodity-production, as it were, from outside of its logic and processes.

Marx's analysis showed that exploitation was inherent in the capitalist system of commodity production, not something perpetrated by cheating, intentional mystification, or purely political clout. Capitalist exploitation is built into the production of commodities when labor itself becomes a commodity. Marx recognized that, even though human beings themselves are reproduced outside the commodity-system, their labor-power is indeed reproduced *by means of* commodities. Labor-power therefore does indeed have a market value *strictu sensu*: its market value – like that of any other commodity, Marx argued – is equal to the value of the commodities required to produce it. Yet its market value, Marx saw, is always *less* than the value that labor-power contributes to production. Thus surplus-value arises from employing labor-power in commodity-production: whatever values may get assigned to non-commodity factors of production, surplus-value is appropriated as the difference between the market value of the goods labor-power produces as output and the market value of the goods required to reproduce it as an input. Market competition then forces capitalists to reinvest appropriated surplus-value in further and/or ever-newer means of production, and that dynamic impels capitalism itself to forever increase in scale, continually drawing more areas of the planet and of human life into the commodity-system.

The crucial question for this view of capitalist production is whether it contains *limits* that are as inherent to its economic dynamic as are exploitation, competition, expansion, and intensification. Marxists have usually argued (in diverse ways) that inherent economic limits to capitalist development *do* exist and therefore that an end to capitalism is historically inevitable.[53] Deleuze and Guattari are not convinced: as we have seen, their view of history (like that of Spinoza, on which in part it is based) is strictly non-teleological. More particularly, they argue that capitalism is able to continually displace any apparent limits to its growth by adding new axioms to its systems of axiomatization. Thus for example when biological and/or political limits appear as obstacles to the extraction of "absolute" surplus-value – a form of surplus-value derived from the brute suppression of wages and/or lengthening of the working day – capital adds axioms of technology to increase productivity within the system of production so that more value (in the form called "relative" surplus-value) can be extracted from the same working day at the same wage-rate. Similarly, when extraction of surplus-value reduces buying-power to the point of threatening a crisis of over-production, axioms of marketing and advertising are added to bolster or fabricate consumer demand. The extension of capitalist axiomatics to global scale, finally, both renews the extraction of absolute surplus-value in some places, and provides additional markets for the redistribution and reappropriation of relative surplus-value, in others. Deleuze and Guattari therefore conclude that the capitalist system of commodity-production has no intrinsic economic limits. It continually *displaces* any apparent limits in the process of expanding and intensifying capitalist production all over the globe.[54]

But what if limits to continued capitalist expansion arise not from within the system of commodity-production (as Marxism has claimed), but from its preconditions, from its relations to what arises outside of its logic – human and natural resources? As the system develops, it must continually draw more of the planet and its populations into commodity-production and consumption; yet those resources are clearly not infinite, and their continued reproduction is by no means guaranteed. In this respect, and as paradoxical as it may sound (given the accounting asymmetry mentioned above), environmental crisis from the perspective of schizoanalysis (and of Bataille) occurs not so much because capitalist society spends too much, but rather because it expends too little while accumulating too much: its "restricted economy" is focused primarily on developing marketable (or "accountable") productive forces, to the detriment of the productive forces of the biosphere as a whole (natural as well as human).[55] At some point, then, the growth imperative of capitalism runs up against the carrying capacity of the planet (Bataille's biosphere): continuous development becomes impossible to sustain.

We are now in a position to better understand Deleuze and Guattari's enigmatic references to the "new earth" as the new socius to follow capital, in the regime of social syntheses we have referred to as "permanent revolution." It should be clear, for one thing, that permanent revolution does not entail continual expansion of the "forces of production," understood in a narrowly quantitative sense as measured by capitalist accounting. For another thing, given the human propensity always to invest in the greater degree of productive force, if capitalist development does indeed exceed the environmental limits of our biosphere and begins to clearly diminish the productive forces of life on the planet, some other relation to the earth may indeed appear "more productive," as was suggested above. Moreover, the invocation of a "new earth" as the fourth socius recalls the socius of savagery, which was the (old) earth. There, death functioned as an experience rather than an "instinct," in alliance- rather than filiation-based relations of anti-production. Of course, lacking the dynamics of market deterritorialization and decoding, savagery was of all the modes of social-production the least free from the repression effected by representation. But the return to alliance-relations, as has been suggested, would free anti-production from the infinite debt and thereby eliminate the socially and psychologically induced need for asceticism and productivism. With the "new earth" as the basis for a more balanced combination of production and anti-production, desiring-production could take full advantage of market decoding without the opposing constraints of capitalist reterritorialization and recoding in the service of the debt.

The new earth can stand, then, for the territory of permanent revolution – a nomadic territory freed from representation, cruelty, terror, and debt by market deterritorialization and decoding. Deleuze and Guattari have insisted from the very beginning of their book that a "schizophrenic out for a walk is a better model than a neurotic lying on the analyst's couch" (2/7), and suggested that "these peregrinations are the schizo's own way of rediscovering the earth" (35/43). This is so not only because schizophrenia epitomizes the legitimate operations of the unconscious but because it at the same time constitutes the ultimate product of capitalism and the true end of universal history.[56] Permanent revolution on the new earth would thus involve a rediscovery of the identity of humankind and nature in a mode of industry no longer driven by debt and favoring instead a new conciliation of social-production with desiring-production.

Feminism and gender

Compared to Marxism and environmentalism, schizoanalysis has relatively little to say about feminism directly, although it does call identity of any kind – including gender identity – radically into question, as we shall see in a moment. Yet the important feminist principle that "the personal is political" resonates with Deleuze and Guattari's insistence that desire and sexuality are directly social despite the prevailing familial representations of them, that desiring-production and social-production are ultimately the same thing, despite the gulf that apparently separates them under capitalism.[57] At the same time, it must be said that the delineation of different modes of social-production and reproduction in Chapter Three of *Anti-Oedipus* raises doubts about the viability of a monolithic concept of "the patriarchy" – a system that would oppress women in the same way regardless of social context. But then again, so do some versions of feminism and gender theory.[58] In any case, that is where our discussion of intersections between schizoanalysis and feminism will begin.

If schizoanalysis had a story to tell about patriarchy, it would be about the becoming-psychological of gender oppression. Whatever the forms of patriarchy instituted in earlier social formations based on codes and over-codes, capitalism has no overarching code by means of which it could impose gender hierarchy on society as a whole. Indeed, capital treats individuals completely indiscriminately, as interchangeable and exchangable quantities of abstract labor. Only subsequent to axiomatization are they endowed with specific skills or tastes to suit them for this branch of production or that field of consumption. So, in principle at least, gender plays little part in the construction of social identity under capitalism. The important exception is the non-remuneration of women's "reproductive" labor, which is one notable feature of the segregation of human reproduction from social reproduction under capitalism that Deleuze and Guattari do not discuss. Controversies over whether such non-remuneration is essential to the extraction of surplus-value from work that is remunerated, or merely a hold-over from older forms of patriarchy and therefore slated for decoding and axiomatization in more advanced stages of capitalism, are not engaged by schizoanalysis. What is clear, however, is that gender was fundamental to social identity under savagery and despotism; there, personal and social identity for the most part coincided, and both were informed by patriarchy.[59] Under capitalism, social identity is abstract or "neuter"; gender hierarchy and personal identity, like despotism (and indeed intimately linked to it, as we shall see), migrate to the heart of the nuclear family and its Oedipus complex. Patriarchy certainly does not disappear under capitalism; it merely goes underground: it becomes psychological rather than socio-cultural or institutional.[60]

Capitalism reproduces patriarchy psychologically by producing hierarchically gendered subjects according to specific mechanisms operating in the nuclear family – mechanisms that, like the Oedipus complex itself, involve the illegitimate use of the syntheses of connection, disjunction, and conjunction. Three polar oppositions form the matrix of nuclear subjectivity: male v. female, object-choice v. identification, and heterosexual v. homosexual. When treated as exclusive disjunctions, these polarities delineate the standardized molar forms of subjectivity that capture and distort desiring-production. Desiring-production itself, of course, treats these oppositions as end-points of a continuum along which desire travels freely, with the result that sex-gender "identity" is actually a polyvalent multiplicity:

> [B]ecause the syntheses constitute local and nonspecific connections, inclusive disjunctions, nomadic conjunctions, [there is] everywhere a microscopic transsexuality, resulting in the woman containing as many men as the man, and the man as many women, all capable of entering – men with women, women with men – into relations of production of desire that overturn the statistical order of the sexes....Desiring-machines [are] the non-human sex: not one or even two sexes, but n sexes....Schizoanalysis is the variable analysis of the n sexes in a subject, beyond the anthropomorphic representation that society imposes on this subject, and with which it represents its own sexuality. The schizoanalytic slogan of the desiring-revolution will be first of all: to each its own sexes.
>
> (295–6/351–2)

Molar representation, by contrast, imposes an exclusive disjunction: the subject must "assume" its sex by choosing either male or female for identification, either male or female for its object-choice, and thus either heterosexuality or homosexuality for its sexual orientation.[6] What is more, with the migration of despotism and paranoia from society at large into the heart of the nuclear family, these intimate patterns of identification, object-choice, and sexual orientation inevitably carry with them investments in either domineering mastery or abject slavery, for as we have seen the only two positions available in the restricted nuclear family when it alone carries the full weight of the "incest-taboo" are those of the castrating despotic father and the tabooed and subjugated mother. The outlines of patriarchal subjectivity are already very clear.

Patriarchal subjectivity originating in illegitimate disjunctive syntheses is then compounded by illegitimate use of the conjunctive synthesis – also operative in racism and nationalism – which produces not just a hierarchically gendered identity but a hierarchical and oppressive value orientation. Segregative (as opposed to nomadic) conjunctions, we have seen, induce in subjects an exclusive sense of superiority in relation to the imputed inferiority of the excluded others. So an Oedipalized subject will, for example, not just identify with the domineering father or heterosexual instead of the subjugated mother or homosexual, but will attribute superior value to domination itself; or conversely, and perhaps just as harmfully, the Oedipalized subject will, after identifying with the subjugated figure, attribute moral superiority to subservience or victimhood itself (as has sometimes been the case with women and homosexuals, and even within feminism[62]). In both cases, the nuclear family produces subjects whose sense of personal identity reproduces patriarchal hierarchies of gender and sexual orientation, even though these hierarchies are not strictly required nor even always reinforced by the more abstract sex/gender-neutral machinery of capitalist social identity.

Where Oedipal gender hierarchies may get reinforced abstractly under capitalism is in the domineering relation of "Mister Capital" to "Madame Earth" (as Marx puts it in *Capital*, to which Deleuze and Guattari add "and their child the Worker" [264/315]). The domination of the earth by capital in social-production is reflected in the domination of the mother by the father in the nuclear family; and, conversely, subjectivity in the nuclear family is perfectly formed to exercise dominion over nature in the capitalist economy. In this respect, it is possible to envisage fruitful intersections of schizo-analysis with both feminism and environmentalism, and thus with ecofeminism.[63] There is reason to doubt, however, that the nuclear family is the only institution capable of producing subjectivity in this way: the homology between the forms of social-production and desiring-production here (as earlier) implies the operation of intermediary forces and practices that would "relay" the abstract machine of domination from one sphere to the other. It may well be that the groups identified by feminism as "masculinist" – authoritarian, competitive, hierarchical, and so on – correspond to those identified by schizoanalysis as subjugated groups, and that the *desiderata* of women's organizational forms – egalitarianism, cooperation, process rather than product orientation, and so on – align them with what Deleuze and Guattari refer to as subject-groups.

In any case, the intersections between feminism and schizoanalysis regarding the role of the nuclear family in reproducing patriarchy suggest at least one concrete practical measure: dissolve the nuclear family. Feminists have long argued that the segregation of the nuclear family from the rest of society warps attitudes toward women (and have called for more egalitarian and socialized child-rearing arrangements, among other things[64]). Schizoanalysis concurs, albeit on somewhat more general grounds: the nuclear family places the mother in a subservient position, as the figure from which children must be weaned by the paternal interdiction, to be sure. But it restricts *all* types of libidinal investment – identification and sexual orientation as well as object-choice – within parameters so narrow that desire not only gets warped but risks getting stifled altogether: asceticism. For schizoanalysis, what is crucial is whether a given type of libidinal investment "engages desire in the Oedipal impasses of the couple and the family in the service of the repressive machines, or whether on the contrary it condenses a free energy capable of fueling a revolutionary machine" (293/349).

The dissolution of the nuclear family by desegregating biological and social reproduction (e.g. integrating child-rearing into wider community relations at work and/or in neighborhoods, housing cooperatives, extended families, etc.) would produce several benefits, from the point of view of schizoanalysis. Socializing reproduction would, for one thing, improve the position of women as mothers and in relation to men: children would not be as desperately attached to one source of nourishment and affection, and would therefore suffer and resent less the process of weaning and the "paternal" interdiction associated with it; the interdiction itself would not be concentrated in one person holding absolute authority (within the family) but would be diffused throughout a broader network of social relations. Perhaps most importantly, more socialized reproduction would sharply reduce the asceticism resulting from the restriction of desire within the nuclear family to precisely those objects that are taboo (parents and siblings): breaking the stranglehold of the nuclear family on desire would enable it to more freely and easily invest social relations at large, thereby breaching the wall between desiring-production and social-production and enabling the former to better saturate and inform the latter.

By multiplying and diversifying the objects and subjects of desire in its formative stages, more fully socialized reproduction would alleviate the rigid bi-polar gender roles produced by the nuclear family thus abetting the propagation of "*n* sexes," as advocated by schizoanalysis. But such proliferation of gender roles and sexual orientations at the same time radically undermines the basis of any "identity politics" for women; ethnic, religious, or racial groups; gays, lesbians, and bisexuals alike. What Deleuze and Guattari say about gay liberation would apply *mutatis mutandi* to feminism and women's movements:

> For example, no "gay liberation movement" is possible as long as homosexuality is caught up in a relation of exclusive disjunction with heterosexuality, a relation that ascribes them both to a common Oedipal and castrating stock, charged with ensuring only their differentiation in two non-communicating series, instead of bringing to light their reciprocal inclusion and their transverse communication in the decoded flows of desire (including disjunctions, local connections, nomadic conjunctions).
>
> (350–1/420)

In the same way, women's liberation is not possible as long as the concept of *woman* itself is not disseminated in a polyvalent multiplicity of different roles and orientations, but remains locked in a bi-polar opposition to man, based on illegitimate uses of the syntheses of connection, registration, and consummation. By contrast, legitimate uses of the syntheses – local part-object rather than global whole-person connections; inclusive rather than exclusive disjunctions; nomadic rather than segregative sedimentary conjunctions – produce subjects that are fluid, ambivalent or polyvalent, open to change; that are continually being made, unmade, and remade.

Such a view of "identity" intersects productively with the gender theory propounded by Judith Butler.[65] Drawing (like Deleuze and Guattari) on Nietzsche as well as on Foucault,[66] Butler brilliantly redefines gender or sexual orientation as an effect of repetition, neither the expression of an inner essence nor the artifact of social construction. Gender norms which are purported to express essential identities are in fact the effect of recurrent acts that constitute them as such.[67] Gender roles are neither the expression of fixed identities nor the result of pure free choice: they stem from the imposition and incorporation of norms in repeated actions and behavior, and have no other ulterior reality than such repetition. However, the constitution of (a sense of) identity by repetition, in Butler's view, is always also subject to variation on that repetition.[68] What repetition may actually produce, as Deleuze also insists, is not just repetition of the same (enforcement of norms) but difference: variation, divergence, deviation, even subversion of norms. The strategic question for Butler is thus "not whether to repeat, but how to repeat or, indeed, to repeat and through a radical proliferation of gender, to displace the very gender norms that enable the repetition itself".[69] By so ascribing a tendentially constitutive yet potentially subversive role to repetition, Butler deftly avoids the conundrum of determinism versus free will and carves out a place for agency in gender theory, with agency now understood in terms of degrees of variation in repetition. Agency is limited but also made possible by repetition.

Agency in repetition for Butler is crucially *ambivalent*, then, in much the same way that the socius and the body-without-organs are under capitalism, according to Deleuze and Guattari. Capitalist axiomatization produces both deterritorialization and reterritorialization; both decoding and recoding; both potential for freedom through differentiation and diversification, and limitations on that potential sponsored by privatized surplus appropriation in the capitalist market and privatized reproduction in the patriarchal nuclear family. The body-without-organs under capitalism, as we have seen, registers desire both to free it from (instinctual or habitual) determination and propel it into new and different trajectories, and to capture it in representations that support existing social power structures. In this connection, schizoanalysis may adduce historical and materialist contexts for the contemporary "gender trouble" that Butler analyzes with such acuity.[70]

Historically, schizoanalysis shows that market decoding destabilizes the symbolic order of culture and therefore undermines personal identity in all of its dimensions, gender and sexual orientation included. The "disorganization

120

and disaggregation of the field of bodies [which] disrupt the regulatory fiction of heterosexual coherence" that Butler refers to is a specific case – indeed a particularly dramatic and highly charged case – of the general dissolution of personal identity effected by axiomatization: persons become mere "images of images," as Deleuze and Guattari put it, even as the number of images increases (with the increase in the number of axioms) and their durability and stability decrease.[71] Furthermore, and paradoxically, even as the nuclear family itself tends to reproduce rigid, bi-polar, gender norms, its enforced segregation from society at large eventually ends up weakening its influence on personal identity: all manner of opportunities for gender displacement, deviation, and subversion become possible in the wide-open spaces outside the family (malls, nightclubs, MTV, etc.) created by market society.[72]

Emerging at the (beginning of the) end of history, the body-without-organs in Deleuze and Guattari's account provides the material basis for the molecular displacement and subversion of identity effected by capitalist deterritorialization and decoding. But it equally registers the forces of molar-paranoid reterritorialization and recoding, ranging from mere herd instinct and conformity (heterosexism and homophobia as fear of difference) to the active enforcement of capitalist and Oedipal asceticism (homophobia as an aversion to sexuality and pleasure in and of themselves). The ambivalence of the body-without-organs thus corresponds precisely to the conception of agency presented by Butler: it is for Deleuze and Guattari the locus of both limitations on and possibilities for difference in repetition.

It would be unfortunate, however, to construe the subversion of identity solely in terms of the historical weakening of constraints on gender and sexual orientation made possible by capitalist decoding. This would be (in a Nietzschean sense) too reactive. Here, Deleuze's materialist ontology of difference intersects very fruitfully with Butler's analysis of subjectivity and repetition. For if agency, as Butler so cogently argues, consists of variation in repetition, and freedom is measured in degrees of variation in repetition, the maximum variation in repetition is precisely what Deleuze and Guattari call schizophrenia. And, as we have seen, schizophrenia designates both the ontological expression of life-force as perpetual differentiation and the potential for freedom made possible, though not fully realized, by capitalism in universal history.

Recapitulation

The process of schizophrenia advocated by schizoanalysis is thus not about going mad or taking merely individual lines-of-flight from institutions of social repression; it is about realizing freedom in difference and through differentiation, the principle of permanent revolution made possible in the universal history inaugurated by capitalism. How do Deleuze and Guattari draw such a conclusion in *Anti-Oedipus*? Basically, by playing Freud, Marx, and Nietzsche off against one another. It may be the structure of the tendentious joke that is most basic to the way the book works: it sets desiring-production and social-production in relation to one another – identity of nature, difference in regime – while at the same time allowing for the historicization and critique of their separation and privatization under capitalism, thereby bringing psychoanalysis as well as political economy to the point of revolutionary autocritique (in the Marxian sense). Furthermore, even though social-production (in characteristically Marxian fashion) determines desiring-production, such determination also allows for historical change, even while the legitimate unconscious syntheses of desiring-production serve as immanent criteria (in the Kantian sense) for the critique of bad psychic organization (the Oedipus, psychoanalysis) and bad social organization (capitalism, the nuclear family) alike.

Yet at the same time, it is Freud who may suffer most from the interference provided by Marx and Nietzsche, since in light of Marxian revolutionary autocritique he is relegated to the company of "bourgeois apologists," like Ricardo and Adam Smith, who reflect merely the apparent objective movement of capitalist society, rather than provide a critique of it. Then again, it is in part the Freudian diagnosis of the Oedipal nuclear family as a breeding-ground for guilt and self-inhibition that enables schizoanalysis to link the critique of capitalist power relations (Father capital, Mother earth, and their child the worker) to Nietzsche's critique of slavish reactivity and asceticism: for it is the nuclear family that produces Oedipally recoded ascetic subjects in the private or domestic sphere, while decoding sponsored by market exchange prevails nearly everywhere else. Conversely, Deleuze and Guattari then extend that diagnosis (via Sartre) to the Oedipal dynamics of subjugated groups, thereby targeting the organizational forms and political strategies of much of traditional Marxism (including most notably the Communist Party), not to mention those of the traditional liberal state. Perhaps it is Nietzsche who comes out least scathed by the interference patterns of the book: his perspective (along with that of Spinoza) grounds the entire historical and psychodynamic process in the unconscious force of life or will-to-power. And yet how far from Nietzschean individualism are the social processes of therapeutic and revolutionary transformation envisioned by schizoanalysis!

The relations between social- and desiring-production are further developed in the homology established between the body-without-organs and the socius, with the forces of production and anti-production that operate in both. This homology is crucially *not* a relation of equivalence, expression, or reflection: the organization of production and anti-production on the socius determines that of the body-without-organs, which appears in its own right, moreover, only under capitalism. Yet the organization of energies and investments on the body-without-organs in turn provides a model of the psyche that in the internal critique of Oedipus serves to identify and critique the five paralogisms which comprise Oedipal psychoanalysis by making systematically illegitimate use of the syntheses of the unconscious. Comparative analysis of the organization of energies and investments on the socius in different modes of socio-libidinal production then shows in the external critique of Oedipus how capitalism has cobbled together those illegitimate uses of the syntheses from previous social formations to construct and impose the Oedipus as the objective lived representation of desire under capitalism, producing ascetic subjects perfectly suited to the demands of the capitalist socius.

Yet the most distinctive feature of the capitalist socius, and of the body-without-organs it fosters, is their *ambivalence*. Deleuze and Guattari mobilize the critique of representation to show how free-form desire gets captured by representations on the socius and body-without-organs alike – even while the capitalist market, with its propensity to deterritorialize and decode, undermines the stability and force of all such representations. Thus, although capitalist axiomatization insistently reterritorializes and recodes in the service of power and the past, it also continually deterritorializes and decodes, providing opportunities for the free-form of semiosis Deleuze and Guattari champion in the name of schizophrenia. So it is that schizophrenia on the body-without-organs emerges at/as the end of universal history as the principle of freedom in permanent revolution.

Yet for schizoanalysis, schizophrenia is not just the principle of permanent revolution: it is also the process of revolution itself. It therefore entails more than individual lines-of-flight from and decodings of the molar representations enforcing exploitation and asceticism under capitalism: it is also the *modus operandi* of subject-groups – whether they be artists, scientists, activists, or whatever – whose very existence and form of operation subvert the dominant mode of organization in power, that of subjugated groups. The chances for realizing permanent revolution, in turn, stem from neither individual lines-of-flight nor the operation of subject-groups occurring in isolation, but from the intersection and assemblage of individuals and groups into a critical mass whose combined effect would be to lift the mortgage of the infinite debt and finally liquidate capital and the barriers it poses to freedom and enjoyment. Permanent revolution, then, is a matter of completing the process of schizophrenia:

> Completing the process and not arresting it, not making it turn in the void, not assigning it a goal....For the new earth...is no more behind than ahead, it coincides with the completion of the process of desiring-production, this process that is always and already complete as it proceeds, as long as it proceeds.

(382/458)

NOTES

1 INTRODUCTION

1 *L'Anti-Oedipe* (1972), the first volume of *Capitalisme et schizophrénie*, was translated into English in 1977. All page references following quotations in the text and notes, except when identified otherwise, refer to the English and then the French editions of this book; all emphases, unless otherwise noted, are the authors' own; also noted are the modifications made to this translation for accuracy or improved clarity and ease of understanding.

2 A few pages from the end of the book, Deleuze and Guattari claim that they "are still too competent; we would like to speak in the name of an absolute incompetence" (380/456). Given the context, they could be referring only to incompetence in the field of psychoanalysis – which itself would belie Guattari's extensive training in and practice of psychotherapy, as well as Deleuze's writings on Freud, especially in *Difference and Repetition* (1994) and *Masochism; an Interpretation of Coldness and Cruelty* (1971); but see also the "willfully incompetent questions" raised on 232/275.

3 These are insistent themes in much of Derrida's work, but see in particular "White mythology" (1974, vol. 6: 5–74) and *Limited Inc.* (1988). Derrida's discursive strategies are distinctive enough for Gregory Ulmer to declare: "Like [Geoffrey] Hartman, I approach Derrida through his style rather than through his philosophical arguments" (*Applied Grammatology* [1985], 318 n. 24); in neither Derrida's nor Deleuze and Guattari's case are style and argument separated to the extent suggested by this offhand statement.

4 Section Five of Chapter One (36–41/43–9) begins by asking: "In what respect are desiring-machines really machines?" and argues that the term desiring-machines is not meant metaphorically; see also 31–3/38–41 and 251–2/299–300. Before collaborating with Guattari, Deleuze (*Difference and Repetition*, 302) had denounced the "bare repetition" of standard conceptual discourse as an inversion and a suppression of true creative ("clothed") repetition:

> Instead of understanding bare repetition as the product of clothed repetition, and the latter as the power of difference, difference itself is made into a by-product of the same in the concept, clothed repetition into a derivative of bare repetition, and bare repetition a by-product of the identical outside the concept.

Before collaborating with Deleuze, Guattari wrote an important essay entitled "Machine and structure" (collected in *Molecular Revolution: Psychiatry and Politics* [1984], 111–19).

5 In a sense, this claim is patently false for Guattari at least, who dealt with schizophrenics in his psychiatric practice at the LaBorde clinic. For more on Guattari and French anti-psychiatry, see G. Genesko (ed.), *The Guattari Reader* (1996). And yet most of the examples of schizophrenics given in the book are characters drawn from art and literature (e.g. Artaud, Beckett), rather than from actual case studies in the narrow sense of the term.

6 Deleuze and Guattari assert that "Our society produces schizos the same way it produces Prell shampoo or Ford cars," adding that "the only difference [is] that schizos are not marketable" (245/292; translation modified).

7 The distinction between schizophrenia and paranoia bears some resemblance to the distinction Lévi-Strauss draws in *The Savage Mind* ([1966], especially at 17) between *bricolage* and engineering. In fact, they explicitly invoke Lévi-Strauss while describing schizophrenic desiring-production:

> The schizophrenic is the universal producer. There is no need to distin-guish here between producing and its product....When Claude Lévi-Strauss defines *bricolage*, he does so in terms of a set of closely interrelated characteristics: the possession of a stock of materials or of rules of thumb that are fairly extensive, though more or less a hodge-podge – multiple and at the same time limited; the ability to continually introduce fragments into new patterns of fragmentation; and as a consequence, a tendency not to distinguish between the act of producing and the product, between the ensemble of instruments to be used and ensemble of results to be achieved.
>
> (7/13; translation modified)

8 In a long passage that Deleuze and Guattari compare with Foucault's view of madness, they quote Laing as saying that "Madness need not be all breakdown. It may also be breakthrough" (131 and 132n./156 and 157n.); see also 362/435.

9 Schizoanalysis would in this respect be a work of *bricolage* in Lévi-Strauss's sense (see note 7, above), inasmuch as it works with what is at hand rather than starting from scratch with a pre-formulated plan. Such a view of philosophical discourse as transformative and creative rather than expository or expressive is laid out in G. Deleuze and F. Guattari, *What Is Philosophy?* (1994). See also note 11 below.

10 To these three figures of central importance to the enterprise, one would want to add Bataille, Bergson, and Spinoza.

11 Deleuze and Guattari insist that they will not play "take it or leave it" with psychoanalysis:

> We see no special problem in the possibility of a coexistence of revolu-tionary, reformist, and reactionary elements at the heart of the same theoretical and practical doctrine. We refuse to play "take it or leave it," under the pretext that theory justifies practice, being born from it, or that one cannot challenge the process of "cure" except by starting from elements drawn from this very cure. As if every great doctrine were not a *combined formation*, constructed from bits and pieces, various inter-mingled codes and flux, partial elements and derivatives, that constitute its very life or its becoming.
>
> (117/139–40)

12 H. Marcuse, *Eros and Civilization: a Philosophical Inquiry into Freud* (1974), especially at 60.

13 To which it would be important to add that in Deleuze and Guattari's view, Marcuse also uncritically retains the concept of sublimation (again moving from the dynamics of authority within the family to society at large, rather than the other way around), and leaves intact Freud's a-historical notion of the "death instinct."

14 See also 29/36–7.

15 See 113/135 and 117/139.

16 Reich's critique of Freud also targets the priority Freud ultimately gave to procreation over polymorphous bodily pleasure, with which Deleuze and Guattari also agree; see 119/141, 291–9/345–7, 331–2/396–7; and also Reich's *The Function of the Orgasm*, especially 282–6.

17 See also 104/124.

18 On cyclical versus linear time, see M. Eliade, *The Myth of the Eternal Return, or, Cosmos and History* (1971).

19 N. O. Brown, *Life Against Death: the Psychoanalytic Meaning of History* (1959), 242; see also 256.

20 Brown, *Life Against Death*,125; see also 171.

21 It is unfortunate that they make no mention of Brown's work; for, along with Ernst Becker's *Escape from Evil* (1975), it the closest thing to an American "equivalent" of *Anti-Oedipus*.

22 Brown, *Life Against Death*, 171 and 242. As Deleuze and Guattari explain:

> [C]astration and Oedipalization beget a basic illusion that makes us believe that real desiring-production is answerable to higher formations that integrate it, subject it to transcendent laws, and make it serve a higher social and cultural production; there then appears a kind of "unsticking" of the social field with regard to the production of desire, in whose name all resignations are justified in advance.
>
> (74/88).

23 Brown, *Life Against Death*, 242 and 19.

24 Brown, *Life Against Death*, 109 and *passim*.

25 See G. Deleuze, *Nietzsche and Philosophy* (1983); and also *Difference and Repetition*, discussed below.

26 Brown, *Life Against Death*, 19.

27 Quoted in A. Mitzman, *The Iron Cage: an Historical Interpretation of Max Weber* (1985), 182; see also Brown, *Life Against Death*, 12.

28 The phrase is from a passage in Marx and Engels' *Communist Manifesto* (in *On Revolution* (1971), 79–107) that informs much of Deleuze and Guattari's understanding of the dynamics of capitalism (and of "decoding" in particular):

> The bourgeoisie cannot exist without constantly revolutionizing the instruments of production, and thereby the relations of production, and with them the whole relations of society....Constant revolutionizing of production, uninterrupted disturbance of all social conditions, everlasting uncertainty and agitation distinguish the bourgeois epoch from all earlier ones. All fixed, fast-frozen relations, with their train of ancient and venerable prejudices and opinions, are swept away, all newly formed ones become antiquated before they can ossify. All that is solid melts into air...
>
> (*On Revolution*, 83)

29 M. Horkheimer and T. Adorno, *Dialectic of Enlightenment* (1972), 44. Although it is beyond the scope of this book, it would be well worth comparing Adorno's "negative dialectics" with Deleuze's poststructuralist philosophy of difference.

30 See G. Lukács, *History and Class Consciousness* (1971).

31 M. Horkheimer and T. Adorno, *Dialectic of Enlightenment*, 7.

32 For a similar argument, see N. Love. *Marx, Nietzsche, and Modernity* (1986). Love's claim, however, is that Marx and Nietzsche are radically incompatible, despite their likenesses; she does not take *Anti-Oedipus* into account.

33 It is my contention that Deleuze and Guattari assign no priority to either social or psychological factors in their critique of modern "ascetic-capitalist" society: the two are interdependent, and must be addressed simultaneously.

34 To which one would want to add the early-modern materialism of Spinoza; on this point see Chapter 4 of this book; A. Negri, *The Savage Anomaly: the Power of Spinoza's Metaphysics and Politics* (1991); and G. Deleuze, *Expressionism in Philosophy: Spinoza* (1990) and *Spinoza: Practical Philosophy* (1988).

35 The three syntheses are discussed in Kant's *Critique of Pure Reason* (trans. F. Max Muller), at A95–A114. Kant introduces the discussion this way:

> [I]t is necessary for us to consider the subjective sources which form the foundation *a priori* for the possibility of experience....If every single representation stood by itself, as if isolated and separated from the others, nothing like what we call knowledge could ever arise, because knowledge forms a whole of representations connected and compared with each other. If therefore I ascribe to the senses a synopsis, because in their intuition they always contain something manifold, there corresponds to it always a synthesis, and receptivity can make knowledge possible only when joined with spontaneity. This spontaneity, now, appears as a threefold synthesis which must necessarily take place in every kind of knowledge, namely, first, that of the *apprehension* of representations as modifications of the soul in intuition, secondly, of the *reproduction* of them in the imagination, and, thirdly, that of their *recognition* in concepts. This leads us to three subjective sources of knowledge which render possible the understanding, and through it all experience as an empirical product of the understanding.

The syntheses of connection, registration, and consommation–consumption play an analogous role for schizoanalysis, except that instead of enabling judgments as to the legitimacy of claims to knowledge, they enable judgments as to the desirability of social formations and representations.

36 Deleuze and Guattari (75/89) explain their recourse to Kant this way:

> In what he termed the critical revolution, Kant intended to discover criteria immanent to understanding so as to distinguish the legitimate and illegitimate uses of the syntheses of consciousness. In the name of *transcendental* philosophy (immanence of criteria), he therefore denounced the transcendent use of syntheses such as appeared in metaphysics. In like fashion we are compelled to say that psycho-analysis has its metaphysics – its name is Oedipus. And that a revolution this time materialist – can proceed only by way of a critique of Oedipus, by denouncing the illegitimate use of the syntheses of the unconscious as found in Oedipal psychoanalysis, so as to rediscover a transcendental

unconscious defined by the immanence of its criteria, and a corresponding practice we call schizoanalysis.

37 Marx in fact credits Engels with having been the one to "call Adam Smith the *Luther of political economy*"; for Marx's discussion of the parallel between Luther and Smith and their insistence on the subjective essence of religious and economic value, see the third manuscript of *The Economic and Philosophical Manuscripts of 1844* (in *Early Writings* [1975], 279–400), especially 341–5. Deleuze and Guattari develop the analogy between libidinal and political economy, linking it with M. Foucault's study of economics and biology (in *The Order of Things: an Archaeology of the Human Sciences* [1994]) this way:

> Michel Foucault has convincingly shown what break (*coupure*) introduced the irruption of production into the world of representation.... Just as Ricardo founds political or social economy by discovering quantitative labor as the principle of every representable value, Freud founds desiring-economy by discovering the quantitative libido as the principle of every representation of the objects and aims of desire. Freud discovers the subjective nature or abstract essence of desire, just as Ricardo discovers the subjective nature or abstract essence of labor, beyond all representations that would bind it to objects, aims, or even to particular sources. Freud is thus the first to disengage desire itself (*le désir tout court*), as Ricardo disengages labor itself (*le travail tout court*), and thereby the sphere of production that effectively eclipses representation. And subjective, abstract desire, like subjective, abstract labor, is inseparable from a movement of deterritorialization that discovers the interplay of machines and their agents underneath all the specific determinations that still linked desire or labor to this or that person, to this or that object, within the framework of representation.
>
> (299–300/356–7; translation modified)

38 For Deleuze and Guattari's understanding of universal history, see 35/43, 139–40/163–4, 153/180, 175–7/207–10, 270–1/322–4, and Chapter 4 of this book.

39 Schizoanalysis makes it possible to situate other figures, too, such as Baudelaire, in such a universal history, as I argue in *Baudelaire and Schizoanalysis: the Sociopoetics of Modernism* (1993); see also my "Schizoanalysis and Baudelaire: some illustrations of decoding at work," in , P. Patton (ed.), *Deleuze: a Critical Reader* (1996), 240–56.

40 As Deleuze and Guattari explain:

> Marx said that Luther's merit was to have determined the essence of religion, no longer on the side of the object, but as an interior religiosity; that the merit of Adam Smith and Ricardo was to have determined the essence or nature of wealth no longer as an objective nature, but as an abstract and deterritorialized subjective essence, *the activity of production in general*. But as this determination develops under the conditions of capitalism, they objectify the essence all over again, they alienate and reterritorialize it, this time in the form of the private ownership of the means of production.
>
> (270/321–2)

41 At the end of the "Introduction" to the *Grundrisse: Introduction to the Critique of Political Economy* (1973), Marx insists: "World history has not always existed; history as world history [is] a result" (110) – i.e. a result of the fact that the abstract category of labor as such "achieves practical truth as an abstraction" only with capitalism (*Grundrisse*, 105).

42 In discussing the relation of bourgeois society and bourgeois "science" to earlier social formations, Marx insists:

> Although it is true...that the categories of bourgeois economics possess a truth for all other forms of society, this is to be taken only with a grain of salt. They [the bourgeois categories] can contain them [aspects of other social forms] in a developed, or stunted, or caricatured form, etc., but always with an essential difference.
>
> (*Grundrisse*, 106)

43 Deleuze and Guattari specify that "capitalism is without doubt the universal of every society, but only insofar as it is capable of carrying to a certain point its own critique – that is, the critique of the processes by which it re-enslaves what within it tends to free itself or appear freely" (270/322). Deleuze and Guattari are no doubt alluding to this passage from the *Grundrisse*, where Marx is again discussing the viability of using contemporary categories to understand previous social formations, here using religious categories as an example: "The Christian religion was able to be of assistance in reaching an objective understanding of earlier mythologies only when its own self-criticism had been accomplished to a certain degree, so to speak, potentially" (*Grundrisse*, 106).

44 They go on to say:

> Universal history is nothing more than a theology if it does not seize control of the conditions of its contingent, singular existence, its irony, and its own critique. And what are these conditions, this point where the auto-critique is possible and necessary? To discover beneath the familial reduction the nature of the social investments of the unconscious.
>
> (271/323)

For further discussion of autocritique in relation to universal history, see 139–40/163–4, 153/180, and 175–7/207–10.

45 On the identity of nature and difference in regime of social- and desiring-production, see 31–2/38–40, 54/63, 99/118, 184/217, and 336–7/402–3, and Chapter 4 of this book.

46 Marx and Engels, *The Communist Manifesto* (see note 28 above).

47 Derrida, it is true, does acknowledge at one point ("Structure, sign, and play in the discourse of the human sciences" [1972], 251) that the priority given to difference arises at a moment that cannot be defined completely in terms internal to the history of philosophy or the human sciences: The moment

> when European culture has been *dislocated*, driven from its locus, and forced to stop considering itself as the culture of reference [in order to confront the play of difference], is not first and foremost a moment of philosophical or scientific discourse, it is also a moment which is political, economic, technical, and so forth.

But these other aspects of the "moment" of European displacement get shorter shrift in Derrida's work than in Deleuze and Guattari's.

48 There are only four mentions of recoding in the entire book (occurring on 135/160, 223/264, 260/309, and 270/322), although its logic is discussed in some detail in relation to reterritorialization, on 221/261, 257/306, and 251/298–9.

49 Even decoding, of considerable importance in *Anti-Oedipus*, virtually disappears in vol. 2 of *Capitalism and Schizophrenia*, whereas deterritorialization becomes even more central and wide-ranging in the second volume; see my "Deterritorializing 'deterritorialization': from *Anti-Oedipus* to *A Thousand Plateaus.*"

50 Alluding to Lacanian usage, Deleuze and Guattari often capitalize the names of the three registers, the Real, the Symbolic, and the Imaginary. Lacan is often alleged to have declared the Real to be "impossible"; what he said was that "the primary process does not meet anything Real other than the impossible" (Lacan, "De mes antécedents," in *Ecrits* [1977]); and that "logic saves us from the Real in order to open access to it in the form of the impossible" (Lacan, "Peut-être à Vincennes," *Ornicar?* [1975], vol. 1). In any case, Deleuze and Guattari's claim that desire produces the Real constitutes a significant departure from this view; they insist at one point that "The real is not impossible..." (27/35).

51 On the secondary counter-production of lack and scarcity, see 28/35–6.

52 At one point, Deleuze and Guattari ask whether psychoanalysis might not be "reviving an age-old tendency to humble us, to demean us, to make us feel guilty" (50/58–9). Later they again ask whether "Transgression, guilt, castration... are determinations of the unconscious, or [rather]...*the way a priest sees things?*" and conclude that by reinforcing feelings of guilt and castration, psychoanalysis merely "invents a last priest" (112/133). (See also 306/365: "we are still pious.")

2 DESIRING-PRODUCTION AND THE INTERNAL CRITIQUE OF OEDIPUS

1 The three syntheses are first described in Sections One through Three of Chapter One; their legitimate and illegitimate uses are then analyzed in Sections Three through Five of Chapter Two, as part of the critique of the Oedipus; finally, they are recapitulated in Section Six of Chapter Two. See also 224/266 and 262/312, where the modes of production are characterized by the type of synthesis that predominates. Deleuze discusses the syntheses extensively in *The Logic of Sense* (1990), 47, 174ff., and 224–34; although they are presented in this earlier work in slightly different terms and a different order, here too the disjunctive synthesis appears to be the most valuable of the three.

2 M. Klein, *Contributions to Psycho-analysis, 1921–1945* (1948). Lacan will incorporate much of Klein's "part-objects" into his notion of the *objet petit-a*; see J. Lacan, *The Four Fundamental Concepts of Psychoanalysis* (1978). Throughout, I use the term "partial-object," in both senses of the word "partial," to underscore that these objects are perceived as partial rather than whole, and partially rather than "objectively": i.e. they are invested with libidinal value; see the English translators' note to this effect (*Anti-Oedipus*, 309). For Deleuze's extensive discussion of partial-objects and their relevance to schizophrenia and the Oedipus, see *The Logic of Sense* (1990), 187–216.

3 Rube Goldberg "machines" furnish a useful illustration of how the connective synthesis works; indeed, two Goldberg drawings appear in the Appendix to the French edition of *Anti-Oedipus* ("bilan-programme pour machines désirantes"), at 464–5.

4 S. Freud, "Note on a mystic writing pad," *The Standard Edition of the Psychological Works of Sigmund Freud*, J. Strachey (ed.) (1966–74), vol. 19: 227–32; J. Derrida, "Freud and the scene of writing," in *Writing and Difference* (1978), 196–231.

5 Shortly after introducing the term "body-without-organs," Deleuze and Guattari quote (9/15) from a poem by Artaud:

> The body is the body
> it is all by itself
> and has no need of organs
> the body is never an organism
> organisms are enemies of the body

Deleuze discusses the body-without-organs in *The Logic of Sense* (at 88–92, and 188–203), in contrast to the views of Melanie Klein. In relation to what Deleuze here calls "counter-actualization" (see *The Logic of Sense*, 150–2, 212, and *passim*), and what Deleuze and Guattari call "anti-production" in *Anti-Oedipus*, the body-without-organs is a locus of freedom.

6 For comparisons of Deleuze's philosophy of difference with that of Derrida, see B. Baugh, "Making the difference: Deleuze's difference and Derrida's differance" (1997) and E. W. Holland, "Marx and poststructuralist philosophies of difference" (1997).

7 For an extensive exploration of the role of repetition in psychic life, see Deleuze's study of sadism and masochism as distinct forms of repetition in *Masochism: an Interpretation of Coldness and Cruelty* (1971).

8 Deleuze discusses the death instinct at some length in *The Logic of Sense* (at 156, 209, 222, and *passim*); for Deleuze's earlier treatment of anti-production, under the name of "counter-actualization," see note 5 above.

9 For Deleuze's discussion of the de-sexualization of energy within the psyche, see *The Logic of Sense*, 208–45, and his *Masochism; an Interpretation of Coldness and Cruelty* (1971).

10 The desirability of the body-without-organs is made clear in a chapter sub-title from *A Thousand Plateaus*: "How to make yourself a body-without-organs" (Plateau Six).

11 For Deleuze's analysis of time and the unconscious, see his *Difference and Repetition* (1994), 70–126, 273–6, and 294–7; for Freud, too, of course, there was no time in the unconscious.

12 On the metonymy of desire, see especially J. Lacan, "The agency of the letter in the unconscious," in *Ecrits* (1977).

13 Indeed, schizophrenia is precisely the condition in which no single code does prevail:

> The schizo has at his disposal his own system of coordinates for situating himself, because first of all he has at his disposal his very own recording code, which does not coincide with the social code, or coincides with it only in order to parody it. The code of delirium or of desire proves to have an extraordinary fluidity. It might be said that the schizophrenic passes from one code to the other, that he deliberately *scrambles all the codes*, by quickly shifting from one to another, according to the questions asked him, never giving the same explanation from one day to the next, never invoking the same genealogy, never recording the same event in the same way...

(15/21; translation modified)

14 On the "unary trait" and Lacan's reading of the Little Hans' episode discussed by Freud, see J. Lacan, *The Four Fundamental Concepts of Psychoanalysis*.

15 Deleuze and Guattari describe the "producing/product identity" as

> an enormous undifferentiated object. Everything stops dead for a moment, everything freezes in place and then the whole process will begin all over again....This imageless, organless body, the unproductive, exists right there where it is produced....It is perpetually reinserted into the process of production....The full body-without-organs belongs to the realm of anti-production; but yet another characteristic of the connective or productive synthesis is the fact that it couples production with anti-production, with an element of anti-production.
>
> (7–8/14–15)

For an account of this transformation of energy in comparison with Freud's views, see G. Deleuze, *Difference and Repetition*, 111–14.

16 For Marx's comments on the senses as active theoreticians, see the third manuscript of *The Economic and Philosophic Manuscripts of 1844* (in *Early Writings* (1975), 279–400), especially 351–4.

17 The existence in French of two terms – *refoulement* and *répression*, usually translated by Hurley *et al.* as psychic and social repression respectively – makes it easier for Deleuze and Guattari to draw these distinctions. *Refoulement originaire* is the French term for primal repression (*Urverdrängung*); it is what makes psychic repression (*refoulement*) possible and thus enables social oppression to "take hold" as repression (*répression*) within the psyche. Following Reich, Deleuze and Guattari insist that social oppression–repression determines psychic repression, even while both are made possible by primal repression. See note 26, below; and *Anti-Oedipus*, 184/217 and 339/405–6; for Freud's own elaboration of the notion of primal repression, see "Inhibition, symptoms, and anxiety" (*Standard Edition*, vol. 20: 87–174), at 94; "Psychoanalytic notes on an autobiographical account of a case of paranoia" [Schreber] (*Standard Edition*, vol. 12: 9–82), where it is referred to simply as "fixation" (at 67); "Repression" (*Standard Edition*, vol. 14: 146–58), at 148; and "The unconscious" (*Standard Edition*, vol. 14: 166–215), at 181.

18 For Deleuze's discussion of catatonia in relation to Klein's "depressive position," see *The Logic of Sense*, 189.

19 Freud mentions on several occasions that "neurosis is, as it were, the negative of perversion"; see "Three essays on sexuality" (*Standard Edition*, vol. 7: 130–243), at 165 and 231; and "Fragment of an analysis of a case of hysteria" [Dora] (*Standard Edition*, vol. 7: 7–122), at 50.

20 As Deleuze and Guattari explain

> the subject is produced as a mere residuum alongside the desiring-machines,...he confuses himself with this third [synthesis] and the residual reconciliation that it brings about: a conjunctive synthesis of consummation in the form of a wonderstruck "So *that's* what that was!"
>
> (17–18/24)

21 And the schizophrenic is the one who lives the enjoyment and suffering of experience most intensely: "Far from having lost who knows what contact with reality, the schizophrenic is closest to the beating heart of reality, to an intense

point identical with the production of the real" (87/104). They then (at 88/104–5) quote Reich, who said that, "with respect to their experiencing of life, the neurotic patient and the perverted individual are to the schizophrenic as the petty thief is to the daring safecracker" (Reich, *The Function of the Orgasm: Sex-Economic Problems of Biological Energy* [1971], at 70).

22 Deleuze and Guattari describe catatonics as those who,

> sickened by...Oedipus, but also by the shoddiness and aestheticism of perversions, reach the wall and rebound against it, sometimes with extreme violence. Then they become immobile, silent, they retreat to the body-without-organs, still a territoriality, but this time totally desert-like, where all desiring-production is arrested, or where it becomes rigid, feigning stoppage: psychosis. These catatonic bodies have fallen into the river like dead weights, immense transfixed hippopotamuses who will not come back up to the surface. They have entrusted all their forces to primal repression, in order to escape the system of social and psychic repression that fabricates neurotics.
>
> (135–6/161)

23 A paralogism is a conclusion reached by means of arguments that violate principles of valid reasoning; Deleuze and Guattari are probably echoing Kant's use of the term in the *Critique of Pure Reason* (the "paralogisms of pure reason," at B399–B432). For expository purposes, I here take them up in an order different from that of Deleuze and Guattari; they treat the paralogism of extrapolation first (73/87ff.), then the paralogism of the double bind (79/94ff.), the paralogism of biunivocal application (101/120ff.), the paralogism of displacement (114/136ff.), and lastly the paralogism of the afterward (127/153ff.).

24 Rather than "signifier," "signified," and "referent," Deleuze and Guattari refer to the "repressing representation," the "displaced represented," and the "repressed representative" – and will conclude that "Oedipus is a factitious product of psychic repression" (115/137).

25 As Deleuze and Guattari insist, "representation is always a social and psychic repression of desiring-production, [though] it should be borne in mind that this repression is exercised in very diverse ways, according to the social formation considered" (184/217); the remaining paralogisms further specify the ways in which Oedipal representation contravenes the logic of the unconscious.

26 This ambivalence is crucial to the functioning of the body-without-organs, for better and for worse; Deleuze and Guattari refer to it at one point as a "coincidence":

> these illusions [those perpetrated by representation] would not take hold if they did not benefit from a coincidence and a support in the unconscious itself that ensures the 'hold.' We have seen what this support was: primal repression [*refoulement originaire*], as exerted by the body without organs at the moment of repulsion, at the heart of...desiring-production. Without this primal repression, a psychic repression in the proper sense of the word [*un refoulement proprement dit*] could not be delegated in the unconscious by the molar forces [of social-production and representation] and thus crush desiring-production.
>
> (339/405–6)

See also 184/217–18.

27 The historical judgment among many practicing psychoanalysts is that such shoring-up is less and less possible, as decoding accelerates and neuroses give way

to character disorders such as borderline conditions; see my *Baudelaire and Schizoanalysis: the Sociopoetics of Modernism* (1993), especially Chapters 6 and 7.

28 S. Zizek, *The Sublime Object of Ideology* (1989); and especially *For They Know Not What They Do: Enjoyment as a Political Factor* (1991).

29 Deleuze and Guattari define "the reactionary unconscious investment" as "the investment that conforms to the interest of the dominant class, but operates on its own account, according to the terms of desire, through the segregative use of the conjunctive synthesis from which Oedipus is derived: I am of the superior race" (105/125);

> [T]here is therefore a *segregative use* of the conjunctive synthesis of the unconscious, a use that does not coincide with divisions between classes, although it is an incomparable weapon in the service of a dominating class: it is this use that brings about the feeling of "indeed being one of us," of being part of a superior race threatened by enemies from outside....Oedipus depends on this sort of nationalistic, religious, racist sentiment, and not the reverse: it is not the father who is projected onto the boss, but the boss who is applied to the father...
>
> (103–4/123)

On the primacy of racist, nationalist, and religious factors relative to their application to the family, see 110–11/131–2.

30 On the mathematical (rather than deconstructive) undecidability of the Oedipus, see 80–1/96.

31 Deleuze and Guattari weigh the relative advantages and disadvantages of the terms "double-impasse," "double-bind" (from Gregory Bateson) and "double-hold" (from Henri Gobard) on 110/131.

32 On the "real" difference between the sexes in Lacan, see *The Four Fundamental Concepts of Psychoanalysis*, especially at 204–5.

33 As Deleuze and Guattari put it:

> everyone is bisexual, everyone has two sexes, but partitioned, noncommunicating; the man is merely the one in whom the male part, and the woman the one in whom the female part, dominates statistically. So that at the level of elementary combinations, at least two men and two women must be made to intervene to constitute the multiplicity in which transverse communications are established – connections of partial-objects and flows: the male part of a man can communicate with the female part a woman, but also with the male part of a woman, or with the female part of another man, or yet again with the male part of the other man, etc....In contrast to the alternative of the "either/or" exclusions, there is the "either...or...or" of the combinations and permutations where the differences amount to the same without ceasing to be differences.
>
> (69–70/82)

For a similar view, see J. Butler, *Bodies that Matter: on the Discursive Limits of "Sex"* (1993), at 93–119, especially 99, 103–4, and 112.

34 And moreover these features, of course, vary culturally, i.e. are differently coded in different cultures.

35 This process parallels the way that money historically detaches itself from a matrix of heterogeneous exchange-relations, based on barter, to become the

universal equivalent for all acts of exchange. This parallel is crucial to the link between desiring-production and social-production under despotism and capitalism, as we shall see in the next chapter. See also J.-J. Goux, *Symbolic Economies: After Marx and Freud* (1990).

36 For Deleuze and Guattari's acknowledgement and critique of Melanie Klein, see 44–5/52–3 and 72/86.

37 Legitimate questions can be raised as to whether this tendency in Lacan is not mitigated or mooted by his style of discourse; Barbara Johnson has argued this point against Derrida's accusation that Lacan remains phallogocentric; see her "The frame of reference: Poe, Lacan, Derrida," in J. Muller and W. Richardson (eds), *The Purloined Poe: Lacan, Derrida, and Psychoanalytic Reading* (1988), 213–51.

38 On the paternal signifier and the Oedipus complex in Lacan, see *The Four Fundamental Concepts of Psychoanalysis* and "On a question preliminary to any treatment of psychosis," in *Ecrits*.

39 See among others N. Chodorow, *Feminism and Psychoanalytic Theory* (1978); J. Mitchell, *Psychoanalysis and Feminism: Freud, Reich, Laing and Women* (1975); and J. Rose, "Introduction" to J. Mitchell and J. Rose (eds.), *Feminine Sexuality: Jacques Lacan and the Ecole Freudienne* (1982).

40 For Lacan's discussion of this schema, see "The seminar on 'The Purloined Letter'," in *The Purloined Poe*; and "On a question preliminary to any Treatment of psychosis," in *Ecrits*.

41 As Deleuze and Guattari explain in a note:

> Lacan's admirable theory of desire appears...to have two poles: one related to "the object small-a" as a desiring-machine, which defines desire in terms of a real production, thus going beyond both any idea of need and any idea of fantasy; and the other related to the "great Other" [*A* in the schema above] as a signifier, which reintroduces a certain notion of lack.
>
> (27n./34n.)

42 This deprivation occurs partly because of the segregation of reproduction and partly, as Marx shows, because of alienation in the sphere of production.

43 On the relations among repression, the constitution of whole persons, and the introduction of lack into psychic economy, see 26/34 and 70/84.

44 See Deleuze, *Nietzsche and Philosophy* (1983); and M. Hardt, *Gilles Deleuze: an Apprenticeship in Philosophy* (1993), at 26–55. The notions of "seeing-as" and "form-of-life" in Wittgenstein play comparable roles; see his *Philosophical Investigations* (1953).

45 Deleuze and Guattari draw explicitly or implicitly on Bataille, Marx, and Spinoza for this view of human-natural relations. See G. Bataille, *The Accursed Share: an Essay on General Economy* (1988); K. Marx, *Economic and Philosophic Manuscripts of 1844*, in *Early Writings* (1975), 279–400, especially at 355); and B. Spinoza, *The Ethics* (1994). On Deleuze and Spinoza, see M. Hardt, *Gilles Deleuze*, 56–111; and J. Butler, *Subjects of Desire: Hegelian Reflections in Twentieth-Century France* (1987), 205–17.

46 On the determination of family relations by social-production and desiring-production, see 99/118.

47 Deleuze and Guattari are unequivocal: "Oedipus is always and solely an aggregate of destination fabricated to meet the requirements of an aggregate of departure constituted by a social formation" (101/120).

48 On the delegation of repression to the family, see especially 120–1/143.

3 SOCIAL-PRODUCTION AND THE EXTERNAL CRITIQUE OF OEDIPUS

1 They refer to "savages, barbarians, and the civilized" [*sauvages, barbares, civilisés*].
2 Deleuze and Guattari will indeed insist that

> If capitalism is the universal truth, it is so in the sense that capitalism is *the negative* of all social formations. It [capitalism] is the thing, the unnamable, the generalized decoding of flows that reveals *a contrario* the secret of all these [other] formations [which operate and survive by] coding the flows, and even overcoding them, rather than let anything escape coding.
>
> (153/180; translation modified)

3 On the sense in which Deleuze and Guattari consider the Oedipus universal, in line with Marx's requirements for a universal history, see especially 175/207.
4 The semantic *combinatoire* was developed by A. J. Greimas to map the logic of relations among terms; see *On Meaning: Selected Writings in Semiotic Theory* (1987).
5 On the theory of acephalous societies, see P. Clastres, *Society Against the State: the Leader as Servant and the Humane Uses of Power among the Indians of the Americas* (1977).
6 In *Anti-Oedipus*, Deleuze and Guattari do not use the term "permanent revolution," but refer instead rather cryptically to a "new earth" as the fourth socius, to follow capital; see Chapter 4 of this book. Deleuze refers to permanent revolution on several important occasions in *The Logic of Sense* (1990); see 49 and 72 especially.
7 But we have to be careful about reading this analogy, and the relations between social investment of the socius and psychic investment of the body-without-organs, in the right way: Deleuze and Guattari ask whether "social investments are secondary projections, as if a large two-headed schizonoiac, father of the primitive horde, were at the base of the socius in general?" They answer that

> We have seen that this is not at all the case. The socius is not a projection of the body-without-organs; rather, the body-without-organs is the limit of the socius, its tangent of deterritorialization, the ultimate residue of a deterritorialized socius. The socius – the earth, the body of the despot, capital-money – are clothed full bodies, just as the body-without-organs is a naked full body; but the latter exists at the limit, at the end, not at the origin.
>
> (281/334)

8 On the historical variability of apparatuses of socio-cultural repression and the differing degrees of affinity between the regimes of social-production and desiring production in general, see 184/217; see also Chapter 4 of this book on the identity of nature and difference of regime between social and desiring-machines under capitalism in particular.
9 Deleuze and Guattari are adamant about avoiding misunderstanding on this point:

We can say that social production, under determinate conditions, derives primarily from desiring-production...But we must also say, more accurately, that desiring-production is first and foremost social in nature, and tends to free itself only at the end....The body-without-organs is not an original primordial entity that later projects itself into different sorts of socius....The social machine or socius may be the body of the Earth, the body of the Despot, the body of Money. It is never a projection, however, of the body-without-organs. On the contrary: the body-without-organs is the ultimate residuum of a deterritorialized socius.

(33/40)

10 However, James O'Connor has recently highlighted the importance of what he calls the "secondary contradiction" of capitalism, operating in the sphere of reproduction, for understanding environmental crisis; see his "Capitalism, nature, socialism: a theoretical introduction" in the inaugural (Fall 1988) issue of *Capitalism, Nature, Socialism*, and the ensuing discussion in subsequent issues. See also Chapter 4 of this book. For a more traditional account, see R. Grundman, *Marxism and Ecology* (1991).

11 This procedure of adding terms to extant dualisms may constitute a Deleuzian equivalent of Derridean "deconstruction"; for a comparison between Deleuze and Derridean deconstruction, see my "Deterritorializing 'deterritorialization': from the *Anti-Oedipus* to *A Thousand Plateaus*" (1991).

12 Deleuze and Guattari credit Nietzsche with having explained the importance of debt:

The great book of modern ethnology is not so much Mauss's *The Gift* as Nietzsche's *On the Genealogy of Morals*. At least it should be. For the *Genealogy*, the second essay, is an attempt and a success without equal at interpreting primitive economy in terms of debt, in the debtor–creditor relationship, by eliminating every consideration of exchange or interest 'à l'anglaise'....[Nietzsche] does not hesitate, as does Mauss, between exchange and debt. (Georges Bataille, motivated by a Nietzschean inspiration, will not hesitate either.)

(190/224–5)

They will go on to show how different yet still crucial are the forms the debt assumes under despotism and capitalism.

13 These are the two modes of "generality" analyzed on the first page of *Difference and Repetition*: "Generality presents two major orders: the qualitative order of resemblances and the quantitative order of equivalences."

14 The savage system of anti-production has been analyzed by Mauss and Bataille, among others; see M. Mauss, *The Gift* (1990); and G. Bataille, *The Accursed Share: an Essay on General Economy* (1988).

15 The appeal for schizoanalysis of Louis Hjelmslev's linguistics and Baruch Spinoza's philosophy becomes clearer in this context: both refuse to grant the necessity of transcendent terms for organizing language and social relations, respectively; on Hjelmslev, see especially 242–3/288–9; on Spinoza, 29/36 and 327/390.

16 Deleuze and Guattari show that in the despotic transformation of primitive debt relations, "money is fundamentally inseparable, not from commerce, but from

137

taxes as the maintenance of the apparatus of the State....In a word, money – the circulation of money – *is the means for rendering the debt infinite*" (197/233–4).

17 On savage and despotic surplus as a surplus-value of code, see 148–50/174–6, 163–4/192–3, 194–6/230–2, and 228/270. For Deleuze's own discussion of the voice from on high, see *The Logic of Sense*, 192–3.

18 On the difference between codes and axioms, see 244–52/295–300.

19 On the "original" axioms of capitalism, see 225–8/266–70.

20 Indeed, Deleuze and Guattari suggest that "the strength of capital resides in the fact that its axiomatic is never saturated, that it is always capable of adding a new axiom to the previous ones" (250/297–8).

21 On capitalism as a surplus-value of flows, see 228–34/270–9.

22 On the way that capital-money in the pursuit of surplus-value alters the relation between production and anti-production by making them immanent, one to the other, see especially 335/400; see also 234–6/279–80 on the roles of advertising, the state, and militarism in the production and realization of surplus-value as an end in itself.

23 For illustrations of the taboo against consuming what one has oneself produced, see 148/173–4.

24 This is the context in which Deleuze and Guattari agree with Jung that "the Oedipus complex signifies something altogether different from itself, and that in the Oedipal relation the mother is also the earth" (162/191).

25 On the relation between the connective and disjunctive syntheses in savage society, see especially 188/222.

26 For the critique of "exchangism" in anthropology, see especially 185/218.

27 Following anthropologists including Griaule, Jaulin, and Adler and Cartry, Deleuze and Guattari conclude that "incest is a pure limit" (160–1/188–9). On the supposed applicability of the Oedipus to pre-modern non-European societies, see 154–84/181–217, especially 157–61/185–90 and 167–72/197–203.

28 On the co-existence of two inscriptions in the imperial social formation, see especially 199/235–6.

29 On the way in which imperial over-coding subsumes savage codes and renders the debt infinite, see 199/236.

30 The representative of desire "eventually" becomes resistance and rebellion because although the law starts out in the service of the despot, it gradually gets appropriated by the masses in an attempt to defend themselves from the despot. For a similarly Nietzschean analysis of the attempt to use state law against the state, see W. Brown, *States of Injury: Power and Freedom in Late Modernity* (1995).

31 The desire for immediate appropriation of life (the repressed representative of desire under savagery) still obtains under despotism but, inasmuch as the despot owns the rights to all life and all means of life, it gets over-coded under despotism and the repressed representative of desire becomes revolt against the despot.

32 Deleuze and Guattari take for granted some familiarity with Marx's analysis of over-production: briefly, the extraction of surplus-value from the circuits of production and sale of commodities leaves the working-class with insufficient purchasing power to buy back the goods they have produced, the result being periodic "crises of over-production."

33 On the capitalist epoch as an age of combined cynicism and piety, see 225/267.

34 See K. Marx, *Capital* (1967), vol. 3: 249–50; see also *Grundrisse: Introduction to the Critique of Political Economy* (1973), 618–23, especially the following (at 623):

In one period the process appears as altogether fluid – the period of the maximum realization of capital; in another, a reaction to the first, the other moment asserts itself all the more forcibly – the period of the maximum devaluation of capital and congestion of the production process.

35 The simultaneity of the two moments does not preclude the possibility that one moment or the other might predominate in a given historical period, or that such predominance might alternate periodically along with business cycles; the 1960s might represent a moment of predominant deterritorialization and decoding, for example, and the 1980s a moment of predominant reterritorialization and recoding. For another example, drawn from the nineteenth century, see my *Baudelaire and Schizoanalysis: the Sociopoetics of Modernism* (1993).

36 For the elaboration of such a definition, see the works of A. Negri, especially *Marx Beyond Marx: Lessons on the* Grundrisse (1984).

37 On the tendency of capitalist inscription to replace qualitative memory and belief with quantified ownership (of either capital or labor-capacity), see 250–1/298.

38 About the transition from despotism to capitalism, Deleuze and Guattari will say: "It is now up to the State to recode as best it can…" (223/264), this being one of the few times that they actually use the term "recode" (see Chapter 1, note 48).

39 In addition to *The Communist Manifesto* (in *On Revolution* [1971]), compare the following passages from *Grundrisse*:

The dissolution of all products and activities into exchange values presupposes the dissolution of all fixed personal (historic) relation of dependence…as well as the all-sided dependence of the producers on one another….The reciprocal and all-sided dependence of individuals who are indifferent to one another forms their social connection. This social bond is expressed in *exchange value*.

(156)

[M]oney as such…[or the] mania for wealth, necessarily bring with it the decline and fall of the ancient communities. Hence it is the antithesis to them. It [money] is itself the community, and can tolerate none other standing above it.

(223)

40 On the development of "true" industrial capitalism from mercantile capitalism, see *Grundrisse*, 250–63.

41 "It is only in the capitalist social formation," Deleuze and Guattari insist,

that the Oedipal limit finds itself not only occupied, but inhabited and lived, in the sense in which the social images produced by the decoded flows actually fall back on restricted familial images invested by desire. It is at this point in the Imaginary that Oedipus is constituted, at the same time as it *completes its migration* in the…elements of representation: *the displaced represented has become, as such, the representation of desire.*

(266–7/317–18)

42 Indeed, Deleuze and Guattari insist that the death instinct becomes an instinct only with capitalism; for under despotism, it was an external threat rather than an internal principle of psychic functioning.

43 For a discussion of loci of recoding in contemporary capitalism, see my "The *Anti-Oedipus*: Postmodernism in Theory" (1988).

44 On the application of the social axiomatic to the nuclear family and the ensuing correlation between "subjective abstract Labor as represented in private property" and "subjective abstract Desire as represented in the privatized family," see 303–4/361–2.

4 BEYOND CRITIQUE: SCHIZOANALYSIS AND UNIVERSAL HISTORY

1 On the splitting of the subjective essence of human life under capitalism into abstract labor and abstract desire, see 337/403.

2 On the identity of nature and difference of regime of desiring-production and social-production, Deleuze and Guattari assert that

> molar social production and molecular desiring-production must be evaluated both from the viewpoint of their identity in nature (*identité de nature*) and from the viewpoint of their difference in régime (*différence de régime*). But it could be that these two aspects, nature and régime, are...actualized only in inverse proportion. Which means that where the régimes are the closest, the identity in nature is on the contrary at its minimum; and where the identity in nature appears to be at its maximum, the régimes differ to the highest degree.
>
> (336/402)

3 For the "fourth and final" thesis of schizoanalysis, see 366/439ff.

4 Paranoia first arises under despotism in connection with the infinite debt; it also characterizes capitalism inasmuch as the latter incorporates the forms and dynamics of despotism in its moment of reterritorialization and recoding, as we saw in Chapter 3.

5 For the "third" and "first" theses of schizoanalysis, see 356/427 and 342/409, respectively; for a discussion of the psychiatric origin of these terms, see 366/439.

6 Deleuze and Guattari's usage of the terms "molar" and "molecular" derives from physics, where molar designates a body of matter considered as a whole as opposed to its component parts (e.g. molecules); see 180–1/213–14 and especially 280–91/333–46; the terms are also linked here with genetics: the unconscious itself is molecular (107–8/128), although it can be captured in representations functioning in the service of molar formations (such as the family). For further discussion of these terms, see B. Massumi, *A User's Guide to Capitalism and Schizophrenia: Deviations from Deleuze and Guattari* (1992), 47–58; and P. Goodchild, *Deleuze and Guattari: an Introduction to the Politics of Desire* (1996), 158–9.

7 On the selective pressure (in the Darwinian sense) exerted by social machines on desiring-machines, see 287–8/342.

8 On autocritique, see Marx, *Grundrisse* (1973), 106; see also M. Foucault, *The Order of Things: an Archaeology of the Human Sciences* (1994), at 255, for a similar view of "continuous" history as a product of capitalism.

9 This is in direct opposition to what is commonly understood as Hegelian universal history.

10 On the relation of the molecularity of the unconscious to DNA, see 290/343.

11 At the same time, the logic of the fourth term suggests that "permanent revolution" would return to an alliance-based network of social relations, for despotism and capitalism are filiation-based: both forms of power impose an infinite debt on society as the basis of unpayable obligation and unending subjugation. A truly "free market" – i.e. a market free of capitalist power – would replace the savage system of cruelty as a system of temporary negotiable alliances and acquittable debts.

12 The permanent yet impersonal threat of death is examined by P. Virilio in *Popular Defense and Ecological Struggles* (1990); other examples include the Cold War and prospect of nuclear Armageddon, but also the more mundane threat of losing one's job.

13 G. Bataille virulently rejects utilitarianism as an instance of such perversion, in *The Accursed Share: an Essay on General Economy* (1988). For Deleuze and Guattari's analysis of the death instinct, see 184/217, 199/236, 213/252, 223/265, 262/312, and 329–37/393–404.

14 It is not a question of simply eliminating the molar, but subordinating it to the molecular; see Chapter 1 of this book on the revolutionary aim of improving social forms' correspondence with the processes of the unconscious.

15 Schizoanalysis may overlap sufficiently with feminism to target capitalist patriarchy along with the Oedipus and asceticism; see below.

16 This pattern in psychoanalysis is linked directly to the double-movement of capitalist axiomatization:

> Capitalism is inseparable from the movement of deterritorialization, but this movement is exorcised through factitious and artificial reterritorializations. Capitalism is constructed on the ruins of the territorial and the despotic, the mythic and the tragic representations, but it reestablishes them in its own service and in another form, as [subjective] images of capital.
>
> (303/360–61)

17 For Foucault's indispensable account of the shift from objective to subjective representation, see *The Order of Things* (1994), 208–11 and 253–6.

18 On the balance between negative and positive, destructive and constructive moments of the schizoanalytic enterprise, see 311/371, 314/374, and 318/379–80.

19 For more on the positive task of schizoanalysis, see 362/434.

20 As Deleuze and Guattari insist: "Revolutionaries often forget, or do not like to recognize, that one wants and makes revolution out of desire, not duty. Here as elsewhere, the concept of ideology is an execrable concept that hides the real problems..." (344/412).

21 Deleuze and Guattari therefore claim (somewhat facetiously, since it would be patently untrue – at least for Guattari, who treated psychotics in the La Borde clinic), in response to the question of whether they "had ever seen a schizophrenic – no, no, we have never seen one" (380/456). For a categorical distinction between the revolutionary potential of schizophrenia as a process and the schizophrenic as a clinical entity, see 379–80/455–6.

22 Deleuze and Guattari insist that schizoanalysis "does not take itself for a party or even a group, and does not claim to be speaking for the masses. No political program will be elaborated within the framework of schizoanalysis" (380/456). Trying to chart a path to (much less cause) revolution would be much like trying to predict the course of evolution: both are based on differentiation ("random

mutation," molecular improvisation) on the genetic level, which produces unforeseeable and contingent results in the context of the (natural or social) environment.

23 Deleuze and Guattari describe this process of subordination as follows:

> Given a socius, schizoanalysis only asks what place it reserves for desiring-production; what generative role desire enjoys therein; in what forms the conciliation between the regimes of desiring-production and social production is brought about, since in any case it is the same production, but under two different regimes; if, on this socius as a full body, there is the possibility of going from one side to another, i.e. from the side where the molar aggregates of social production are organized to this other side, no less collective, where the molecular multiplicities of desiring-production are formed; whether and to what extent such a socius can endure the reversal of power such that desiring-production subjugates social production and yet does not destroy it, since it is the same production working under the difference in regime...
>
> (380/456–57)

This is, as I have suggested, the Kantian moment of schizoanalysis, where epistemological critique is transformed into revolutionary mobilization.

24 Deleuze and Guattari are clear on the primacy of libidinal force:

> If we wonder where these forms of *force* come from, it is evident that they are not to be explained in terms of any goal or end, since they are what determines goals and ends. The form or quality of a given socius – the body of the earth, the body of the despot, the body of capital – depends on a state or degree of intensive development of productive forces...
>
> (343/410–11)

See also the following crucial formulation: "Libidinal investment does not bear on the regime of the social syntheses, but upon the degree of development of the forces or the energies on which these syntheses depend" (345/413).

25 They prefer "preconscious" to "conscious" interest in this context, because objective interests are not always (are perhaps only rarely) conscious, even though they can be brought to consciousness (which is one of the essential goals of any "vanguard" party).

26 The sources of this view include Spinoza and Bataille as well as Nietzsche; see G. Deleuze, *Nietzsche and Philosophy* (1983); B. Spinoza, *The Ethics* (1994); and G. Bataille, *The Accursed Share* (1994); see also M. Hardt, *Gilles Deleuze: an Apprenticeship in Philosophy* (1993); and J. Butler, *Subjects of Desire: Hegelian Reflections in Twentieth-Century France* (1987).

27 Think for example of the way subversive subcultural forms like rap music get taken up by the music industry, and their subversive potential eventually accommodated to the imperatives of marketing and profit-maximization.

28 On the sheer libidinal pleasures of working for capital, see 346–7/415.

29 On the relations of desire to successful (i.e. permanent) and failed (or recuperated) revolutions, see 377/452.

30 On the actualization of revolutionary potential in a moment of rupture, see 378/453.

31 In Sartre, see especially *The Critique of Dialectical Reasoning*, vol. I: Book I, Part D; and Book II, Part A. Acknowledging their debt to Sartre, Deleuze and Guattari say:

> Sartre's analysis in *Critique de la raison dialectique* appears to us profoundly correct where he concludes that there does not exist any class spontaneity, but only a "group" spontaneity: whence the necessity for distinguishing "groups-in-fusion" from the class, which remains "serial," represented by the party or the State.
>
> (256–7/305)

See also 64/75–6, 277/329, 348–9/417–18, 377/452–3. Although Guattari published relatively little prior to collaborating with Deleuze, he discusses his debts to Sartre in an essay entitled "The group and the person" (collected in *Molecular Revolution: Psychiatry and Politics* [1984], 24–44), especially 27.

32 Similarly, a given individual (Deleuze and Guattari instance Saint-Juste and Lenin) can participate in both kinds of group at different times; see 349/418.

33 Deleuze and Guattari explain that

> there is first a real libidinal [unconscious] revolutionary break, which then shifts into the position of a simple [preconscious] revolutionary break with regard to aims and interests, and finally re-forms a merely specific reterritoriality, a specific body on the full body of capital. Subjugated groups are continually deriving from subject-groups. One more axiom.
>
> (375/450)

34 On the differences between strategy and tactics, see M. de Certeau, *The Practice of Everyday Life* (1984); de Certeau draws on Von Clausewitz.

35 But for a more nuanced discussion of sports and schizoanalysis, see my "'Introduction to the non-fascist life': Deleuze and Guattari's 'revolutionary' semiotics" (1987).

36 On the way paranoiacs apply to the family an originally social delirium (of "races, ranks, classes, and universal history"), see 365/438.

37 All it takes for the molar-paranoid type of investment informing subjugated groups to develop into full-fledged fascism, as I have argued elsewhere, is for these "intermediary institutions" to congeal around a common political authority-figure, thereby forming a central sovereignty; ordinarily, the market system keeps them relatively autonomous from one another, under what I have here called the neo-sovereignty of capital. See Foucault's "Preface" to the English edition of *Anti-Oedipus* and my "Introduction to the non-fascist life" (1987). See also note 39, below, on the "specifically artistic Oedipus" and the "specifically scientific Oedipus" imposed by the state on these group activities.

38 Deleuze and Guattari insist that the Oedipus is more than a family structure: it is also

> a means of integration into the group,...[For] Oedipus flourishes in subjugated groups, where an established order is invested through the group's own repressive forms. And it is not the forms of the subjugated group that depend on Oedipal projections and identifications, but the reverse: it is Oedipal applications that depend on the determinations of

the subjugated group as an aggregate of departure and on their libidinal investments.

(103/123)

39 On Deleuze and Guattari's appeals to art and science as more or less pure experimentation, and therefore *potentially* revolutionary, see 368–71/442–5 and 379/454–5. Deleuze and Guattari develop their views on the relations among philosophy, art, and science in *What Is Philosophy?* (1994); see especially Part Two.

40 One of the key paradoxes of schizoanalysis is that desire both desires to be free (free-form schizophrenia) yet also desires greater force (development of productive force): only the elimination of power from capitalism promises the realization of *both* greater force and greater freedom – which is why this mode of production stands at the threshold of universal history, according to Deleuze and Guattari.

41 Although humankind, because of its "productive capacities," does tend to develop life-force to a greater degree than most other species on the planet – for better and for worse. See *The Accursed Share* for Bataille's account of the way all life-forms (species) seek to expand their force to the utmost allowed by the environment.

42 A. Negri, *Marx Beyond Marx: Lessons on the Grundrisse* (1984); and *The Politics of Subversion: a Manifesto for the Twenty-First Century* (1989). Negri was imprisoned for being a spokesman and theorist for the *autonomia* movement in Italy, and was strongly supported by Deleuze, who wrote a preface to the French translation of his book on Spinoza (*The Savage Anomaly: the Power of Spinoza's Metaphysics and Politics* [1991]). For further reflections on Marxism along the lines presented in *Anti-Oedipus*, see Guattari and Negri's *Communists Like Us: New Spaces of Liberty, New Lines of Alliance* (1990).

43 See J. Butler, *Subjects of Desire*, 205 and *passim*; and M. Hardt, *Gilles Deleuze*, 72, 93 and *passim*.

44 For a survey of philosophies of history in Marx, see W. Adamson, "Marx's four histories: an approach to his intellectual development," *History and Theory* (1982). Rather than search for a definitive "break" separating distinct positions in Marx (as Althusser does for Marx, and Negri for Spinoza), it seems to me more rigorous and fruitful to recognize tensions within the corpus among different or "competing" views; see, for an example, E. Balibar, *The Philosophy of Marx* (1995). On Spinoza's possible influence on Marx (who hand-copied whole passages from the *Tractatus Theologico-Politicus*), see the articles in *Cahiers Spinoza* (1977), vol. 1, by M. Rubel ("Marx à la rencontre de Spinoza," 7–28), A. Matheron ("Le *Traité Théologico-Politique* vu par le jeune Marx," 159–212), and A. Igoin ("De l'ellipse de la théorie politique de Spinoza chez le jeune Marx," 213–28); this issue also reprints in their entirety the passages Marx hand-copied from Spinoza.

45 Forces of production include the labor-power of the proletariat, to be sure, but also the knowledge, technology, and organization provided by the capitalist; relations of production include the relations between the classes, clearly, but also cultural or ideological elements (such as possessive individualism or asceticism) which may be common to both workers and capitalists, yet serve neither's interests. For attempts to construe class in other than transcendental-subjective terms, see N. Poulantzas, *Classes in Contemporary Capitalism* (1975); and G. Carchedi, *On the Economic Identification of Social Classes* (1977).

46 This model appears in K. Marx and F. Engels, *The Communist Manifesto*:

> At a certain stage of the development of [the] means of production and of exchange, the conditions under which feudal society produced and exchanged...became no longer compatible with the already developed productive forces; they became so many fetters. They had to be burst asunder; they were burst asunder.
>
> (*On Revolution*, 84–5)

Here history as class struggle nevertheless also appears, in one of its most striking formulations: "The history of all hitherto existing society is the history of class struggles" (81). One of Marx's key moves was of course to replace Hegel's subject–object dialectic of Spirit and Matter with a dialectic between transformative human labor and the natural environment. But such a "materialist" reversal of Hegel may end up merely producing a Marxian "metaphysics of production" (see for example J. Baudrillard, *The Mirror of Production* [1975]), and/or merely reproducing a subject–object dialectic in which the fate of the human species is irrevocably tied to the domination of nature. In any case, the presumption that the development of productive force would in and of itself produce human freedom appears increasingly dubious: already in the 1950s, Marcuse (in *Eros and Civilization: a Philosophical Inquiry into Freud* [1955; 1974]) coined the important term "surplus-repression" to designate the lag between the development of productive forces and the realization of freedom; more recently, Régis Debray (in *Critique of Political Reason* [1983]) has gone so far as to deny any link whatsoever between the development of productive forces and the prospects for political advancement and the realization of freedom.

47 Most notably in his "Critique of the Gotha Program" (*On Revolution*, 488–506), where Marx insists that value derives from nature as well as from human labor; see also the passages on alienation in "The economic and philosophical manuscripts of 1884" (*Early Writings* [1975], 279–400, especially 324–7 and 354–8), where he asserts that humankind is part of nature.

48 Very early in the book, Deleuze and Guattari explain that they

> make no distinction between man and nature: the human essence of nature and the natural essence of man become one within nature in the form of production or industry, just as they do within the life of man as a species. Industry is then no longer considered from the extrinsic point of view of utility, but rather from the point of view of its fundamental identity with nature as production of man and by man. Not man as the king of creation, but rather as the being who is in intimate contact with the profound life of all forms or all types of beings...
>
> (4/10)

For a very useful application of this view to questions of modernity, science, and epistemology, see B. Latour, *We Have Never Been Modern* (1993), 117, 125, and *passim*.

49 On Spinoza and environmentalism, see A. Ness, "Spinoza and ecology," in *Speculum Spinozanum, 1677–1977* (1977), 418–25, where he asserts that "No great philosopher has so much to offer in the way of clarification and articulation of basic ecological attitudes as Baruch Spinoza" (423). See also his *Freedom, Emotion and Self-Subsistence* (1975); and A. Collier, "The inorganic body and the ambiguity of freedom," *Radical Philosophy* (1991).

50 Deleuze and Guattari are most explicit about their debt to Spinoza: "The body-without-organs is the immanent substance, in the most Spinozist sense of the

word; and the partial objects are like its ultimate attributes" (327/390); but see also 309n./369n., and in a more political context, 29/36.

51 For similar views, see N. O. Brown, *Life Against Death: the Psychoanalytic Meaning of History* (1959); and M. Horkheimer and T. Adorno, *Dialectic of Enlightenment* (1972).

52 This helps explain the controversies surrounding the relation of the sphere of reproduction to that of production, and the difficulties of subsuming education and even job training into capitalist accounting.

53 But consider Marx on the law of the counteracted tendency: the tendency of the rate of surplus-value is to fall (with the increasing proportion of constant to variable capital), but that tendency is counteracted by the growth of surplus-value in quantitative terms (due notably to the shift from absolute to relative surplus-value).

54 On the displacement of limits under capitalism, see 175–7/207–9, 231/275, 245–7/291–4, and 266–7/317–19.

55 In addition to *The Accursed Share*, see Bataille's earlier (1933) essay entitled "The notion of expenditure," in *Visions of Excess: Selected Writings, 1927–1939* (1985), 116–29.

56 On schizophrenia as the absolute limit of capitalism (which is itself the relative limit of all other societies), see 2–5/7–11, 35/43, and 130–1/155. For Guattari's own subsequent reflections on environmentalism, see his *Les trois écologies* (1989).

57 For Deleuze and Guattari's insistence on the thoroughly social quality of all interpersonal relations, see 293–4/349, and 357/428. With the important exceptions of Judith Butler (who draws on *Difference and Repetition*, as discussed below) and Kathi Weeks (who draws on *Nietzsche and Philosophy* in her "Subject for a feminist standpoint," *Marxism Beyond Marxism* [1996]), most feminist responses to Deleuze and Guattari have not addressed schizoanalysis, but rather the concept of "becoming-woman" presented in *A Thousand Plateaus*, discussion of which lies beyond the scope of the present work; see for example the section of C. Boundas and D. Olkowski's *Gilles Deleuze and the Theater of Philosophy* (1994) devoted to "The question of becoming-woman," which includes essays by R. Braidotti ("Toward a new nomadism: feminist Deleuzian tracks; or, metaphysics and metabolism") and E. Grosz ("A thousand tiny sexes: feminism and rhizomatics"); and C. Griggers, *Becoming-Woman* (1997). Among the most significant feminist responses to Deleuze and Guattari are A. Jardine, *Gynesis: Configurations of Woman and Modernity* (1985), Chapter 10; R. Braidotti, *Patterns of Dissonance: a Study of Women in Contemporary Philosophy* (1991), Chapters 3 and 5, and *Nomadic Subjects: Embodiment and Sexual Difference in Contemporary Feminist Theory* (1994), "Introduction" and Chapter 5; and E. Grosz, *Volatile Bodies: Toward a Corporeal Feminism* (1994), Chapter 7, and *Space, Time, and Perversion: Essays on the Politics of Bodies* (1995), Chapter 13.

58 See for example J. Butler, *Gender Trouble: Feminism and the Subversion of Identity* (1990), 1–6 and *passim*.

59 Although it is well beyond the scope of this book, further schizoanalysis of the patriarchies of savagery and despotism would show that they operate very differently.

60 To say that under capitalism patriarchy is *primarily* psychological rather than institutional does not mean that capitalist institutions are not patriarchal – far from it. It means rather that the myriad ways patriarchy gets reproduced under capitalism (including within institutions) are not intrinsic to axiomatization, but

derive from processes of reterritorialization and recoding. To illustrate the point a different way: the most virulent forms of homophobia, gay-bashing for example, are psychologically rather than institutionally motivated, even though homophobia may permeate institutional cultures as well (in other, perhaps milder, forms).

61 For illuminating analyses of how the Oedipus suppresses homosexuality even more severely and effectively than it does incest, see J. Butler, *Gender Trouble*, especially 72–88; and *Bodies that Matter: on the Discursive Limits of "Sex"* (1993), especially 93–119. The act of assuming a bipolar sexual identity is central to Lacanian accounts of subjectivity.

62 See W. Brown's critiques of victimhood and identity politics in *States of Injury: Power and Freedom in Late Modernity* (1995).

63 For an analytic survey of ecofeminism, see C. Merchant, *Radical Ecology: the Search for a Liveable World* (1992), 183–210; for a sample of the field, see anthologies by K. Warren; see also D. Haraway, *Simians, Cyborgs, and Women: the Reinvention of Nature* (1991); and N. Sturgeon, *Ecofeminist Natures: Race, Gender, Feminist Theory, and Political Action* (1997).

64 See for example N. Chodorow, *The Reproduction of Mothering: Psychoanalysis and the Sociology of Gender* (1978); and D. Dinnerstein, *The Mermaid and the Minotaur: Sexual Arrangements and Human Malaise* (1976).

65 See J. Butler, *Gender Trouble* and *Bodies that Matter*.

66 See her Nietzschean critique of Lacan's "religious idealization of failure":

> Lacanian theory must be understood as a kind of "slave morality." How would Lacanian theory be reformulated after the appropriation of Nietzsche's insight in *On the Genealogy of Morals* that God, the inaccessible Symbolic, *is rendered inaccessible* by a power (the will-to-power) that regularly institutes its own powerlessness [in the form of nihilism]? This figuration of the paternal law as the inevitable and unknowable authority before which the sexed subject is bound to fail must be read for the theological impulse that motivates it as well as for the critique of theology that points beyond it. The construction of the law that guarantees failure is symptomatic of a slave morality that disavows the very generative powers it uses to construct the "Law" as a permanent impossibility.
>
> (Butler, *Gender Trouble*, 57)

See also her Foucauldian critique of psychoanalysis: "the desire which is conceived as both original and repressed is the effect of the subjugating law itself" (ibid., 65). Both of Butler's critiques intersect with Deleuze and Guattari's own.

67 "There is no gender identity behind the expressions of gender; that identity is performatively constituted by the very 'expressions' that are said to be its results" (Butler, *Gender Trouble*, 25).

68 ibid., 145 and *passim*.

69 *Gender Trouble*, 148. Compare this with what Deleuze has to say about "counter-actualization" as the force of freedom in and through repetition:

> Counter-actualization is nothing, it belongs to a buffoon when it operates alone and pretends to have the value of *what could have happened*. But, to be the mime of *what effectively occurs*, to double the actualization with a counter-actualization, the identification with a distance, like

the true actor and dancer, is to give to the truth of the event the only chance of not being confused with its inevitable actualization.

(*The Logic of Sense*, 161)

70 Such contextualization intersects with Butler's repeated calls for the historicization of the Lacanian "Symbolic Order"; see *Gender Trouble*, 66, 73, 76 and *passim*.

71 ibid., 136.

72 John D'Emilio has made perhaps the most explicit case for the contributions of capitalism to the emergence of viable gay and lesbian identities, for example, which he attributes to the weakening of family and conjugal influences in the face of increasing socialization of production and leisure; see his *Making Trouble: Essays on Gay History, Politics, and the University* (1992), especially "Capitalism and gay identity," 3–16.

BIBLIOGRAPHY

Adamson, W., "Marx's four histories: an approach to his intellectual development," *History and Theory*, 1982, vol. 20: 379–402.

Balibar, E., *The Philosophy of Marx*, trans. C. Turner, New York: Verso, 1995.

Bataille, G., *Visions of Excess: Selected Writings, 1927–1939*, A. Stoekl (ed.), Minneapolis: University of Minnesota Press, 1985.

—— *The Accursed Share: an Essay on General Economy*, trans. R. Hurley, New York: Zone Books, 1988.

Baudrillard, J., *The Mirror of Production*, trans. M. Poster, St Louis: Telos Press, 1975.

Baugh, B., "Making the difference: Deleuze's difference and Derrida's differance," *Social Semiotics*, 1997, vol. 7: 127–49.

Becker, E., *Escape from Evil*, New York: Free Press, 1975.

Bey, H., *T.A.Z.: the Temporary Autonomous Zone, Ontological Anarchy, Poetic Terrorism*, Brooklyn, NY: Autonomedia, 1991.

Boundas, C. and Olkowski, D. (eds), *Gilles Deleuze and the Theater of Philosophy*, New York: Routledge, 1994.

Braidotti, R. *Patterns of Dissonance: a Study of Women in Contemporary Philosophy*, trans. E. Gould, Cambridge: Polity Press, 1991.

—— *Nomadic Subjects: Embodiment and Sexual Difference in Contemporary Feminist Theory*, New York: Columbia University Press, 1994.

—— "Toward a new nomadism: feminist Deleuzian tracks; or, metaphysics and metabolism" in C. Boundas and D. Olkowski (eds), *Gilles Deleuze and the Theater of Philosophy*, 159–86.

Brown, N. O., *Life Against Death: the Psychoanalytic Meaning of History*, Middletown: Wesleyan University Press, 1959.

Brown, W., *States of Injury: Power and Freedom in Late Modernity*, Princeton, NJ: Princeton University Press, 1995.

Butler, J., *Subjects of Desire: Hegelian Reflections in Twentieth-Century France*, New York: Columbia University Press, 1987.

—— *Gender Trouble: Feminism and the Subversion of Identity*, New York: Routledge, 1990.

—— *Bodies that Matter: on the Discursive Limits of "Sex"*, New York: Routledge, 1993.

Carchedi, G., *On the Economic Identification of Social Classes*, London: Routledge & Kegan Paul, 1977.

—— *Class Analysis and Social Research*, Oxford: Blackwell, 1987.

Certeau, M. de., *The Practice of Everyday Life*, trans. S. Rendall, Berkeley: University of California Press, 1984.

Chodorow, N., *The Reproduction of Mothering: Psychoanalysis and the Sociology of Gender*, Berkeley: University of California Press, 1978.

—— *Feminism and Psychoanalytic Theory*, New Haven, CT: Yale University Press, 1989.

Clastres, P., *Society Against the State: the Leader as Servant and the Humane Uses of Power among the Indians of the Americas*, trans. R. Hurley, New York: Urizen Books, 1977.

Collier, A., "The inorganic body and the ambiguity of freedom," *Radical Philosophy*, 1991, vol. 57: 3–9.

D'Emilio, J. *Making Trouble: Essays on Gay History, Politics, and the University*, New York: Routledge, 1992.

Debray, R., *Critique of Political Reason*, trans. D. Macey, London: Verso, 1983.

Deleuze, G. *Masochism; an Interpretation of Coldness and Cruelty*, trans. J. McNeil, New York: G. Braziller, 1971.

—— *Nietzsche and Philosophy*, trans. H. Tomlinson, New York: Columbia University Press, 1983.

—— "The group and the person," collected in F. Guattari, *Molecular Revolution: Psychiatry and Politics* (1984), 24–44.

—— *Spinoza, Practical Philosophy*, trans. R. Hurley, San Francisco: City Lights Books, 1988.

—— *Expressionism in Philsophy: Spinoza*, trans. M. Joughin, New York: Zone Books; Cambridge, MA: MIT Press, 1990.

—— *The Logic of Sense*, trans. M. Lester with C. Stivale, New York: Columbia University Press, 1990.

—— *Difference and Repetition*, trans. P. Patton, New York: Columbia University Press, 1994.

Deleuze, G. and F. Guattari, *L'Anti-Oedipe: capitalisme et schizophrénie*, nouvelle édition augmente, Paris: Minuit, 1972 (includes the essay "Bilan-programme pour machines désirantes" as an appendix).

—— *Anti-Oedipus: Capitalism and Schizophrenia*, trans. R. Hurley, M. Seem, and H. Lane, Minneapolis: University of Minnesota Press, 1977.

—— *A Thousand Plateaus: Capitalism and Schizophrenia*, trans. B. Massumi, Minneapolis: University of Minnesota Press, 1987.

—— *What is Philosophy?*, trans. H. Tomlinson and G. Burchell, New York: Columbia University Press, 1994.

Derrida, J., "Structure, sign, and play in the discourse of the human sciences," in R. Macksey and E. Donato (eds), *The Structuralist Controversy: the Languages of Criticism and the Sciences of Man*, 247–72.

—— "White mythology," *New Literary History*, 1974, vol. 6: 5–74.

—— *Writing and Difference*, trans. A. Bass, Chicago: University of Chicago Press, 1978.

—— *Limited Inc.*, Evanston, Northwestern University Press, 1988 (contains the essays "Signature, event, context" and "Reiterating the differences," from *Glyph* vols 1 and 2).

Dinnerstein, D., *The Mermaid and the Minotaur: Sexual Arrangements and Human Malaise*, New York: Harper & Row, 1976.

Eliade, M., *The Myth of the Eternal Return, or Cosmos and History*, trans. W. R. Trask, Princeton, NJ: Princeton University Press, 1971.

D'Emilio, J., *Making Trouble: Essays on Gay History, Politics, and the University*, New York: Routledge, 1992.

Engels, F., *The Origin of the Family, Private Property, and the State in the Light of the Researches of Lewis H. Morgan*, trans. E. Untermann, New York: International Publishers, 1972.

Foucault, M., *The Order of Things: an Archaeology of the Human Sciences*, New York: Vintage Books, 1994.

Freud, S., *The Standard Edition of the Psychological Works of Sigmund Freud*, J. Strachey (ed.), 24 vols, London: Hogarth Press, 1966–74 (includes *Jokes and their Relation to the Unconscious* (vol. 8), and *Beyond the Pleasure Principle* (vol. 18).

Genesko, G. (ed.), *The Guattari Reader*, Oxford: Blackwell, 1996.

Goodchild, P., *Deleuze and Guattari: an Introduction to the Politics of Desire*, London and Thousand Oaks, CA: Sage, 1996.

Goux, J.-J., *Symbolic Economies: After Marx and Freud*, trans. J. C. Gage, Ithaca, NY: Cornell University Press, 1990.

Greimas, A. J., *On Meaning: Selected Writings in Semiotic Theory*, trans. P. J. Perron and F. H. Collins, Minneapolis: University of Minnesota Press, 1987.

Griggers, C., *Becoming-Woman*, Minneapolis: University of Minnesota Press, 1997.

Grosz, E., *Volatile Bodies: Toward a Corporeal Feminism*, Bloomington: Indiana University Press, 1994.

—— *Space, Time, and Perversion: Essays on the Politics of Bodies*, New York: Routledge, 1995.

—— "A thousand tiny sexes: feminism and rhizomatics," in C. Boundas and D. Olkowski (eds), *Gilles Deleuze and the Theater of Philosophy*, New York: Routledge, 187–210.

Grundman, R., *Marxism and Ecology*, Oxford: Oxford University Press, 1991.

Guattari, F., *Molecular Revolution: Psychiatry and Politics*, trans. R. Sheed, New York: Penguin, 1984 (contains an introductory essay, "The group and the person," by Deleuze).

—— *Les trois écologies*, Paris: Galilée, 1989.

Guattari, F. and Negri, A., *Communists Like Us: New Spaces of Liberty, New Lines of Alliance*, trans. M. Ryan, New York: Semiotext(e), 1990.

Haraway, D., *Simians, Cyborgs, and Women: the Reinvention of Nature*, New York: Routledge, 1991.

Hardt, M., *Gilles Deleuze: an Apprenticeship in Philosophy*, Minneapolis: University of Minnesota Press, 1993.

Hjelmslev, L., *Prolegomena to a Theory of Language*, trans. F. J. Whitfield, Madison: University of Wisconsin Press, 1961.

Hjelmslev, L. and Uldall, H. J., *Outline of Glossematics: a Study in the Methodology of the Humanities, with Special Reference to Linguistics*, Copenhagen: Nordisk Sprog-og Kulturforlag, 1957.

Holland, E. W., "'Introduction to the non-fascist life': Deleuze and Guattari's 'revolutionary' semiotics," *L'esprit créateur*, 1987, vol. 27: 19–29.

—— "The *Anti-Oedipus*: postmodernism in theory, or the post-Lacanian historical contextualization of psychoanalysis," *Boundary 2*, 1988, vol. 14: 291–307.

—— "Deterritorializing 'deterritorialization': from the *Anti-Oedipus* to *A Thousand Plateaus*," *SubStance*, 1991, vol. 66: 55–65.

—— *Baudelaire and Schizoanalysis: the Sociopoetics of Modernism*, Cambridge: Cambridge University Press, 1993.

—— "Schizoanalysis and Baudelaire: some illustrations of decoding at work," in P. Patton (ed.), *Deleuze: a Critical Reader*, Oxford: Blackwell, 1996, 240–56.

—— "Marx and poststructuralist philosophies of difference," *South Atlantic Quarterly*, 1997, vol. 96: 83–96.

Horkheimer, M. and Adorno, T., *Dialectic of Enlightenment*, trans. J. Cumming, New York: Herder & Herder, 1972.

Igoin, A., "De l'ellipse de la théorie politique de Spinoza chez le jeune Marx," *Cahiers Spinoza*, 1977, vol. 1: 213–28.

Jardine, A., *Gynesis: Configurations of Woman and Modernity*, Ithaca, NY: Cornell University Press, 1985.

Klein, M. *Contributions to Psycho-Analysis, 1921–1945*, London: Hogarth Press, 1948.

Lacan, J., "Peut-être à Vincennes" *Ornicar?*, vol. 1, 1975.

—— *Ecrits*, trans. A. Sheridan, New York: Norton, 1977.

—— *The Four Fundamental Concepts of Psychoanalysis*, trans. A. Sheridan, New York: Norton, 1978.

—— *Feminine Sexuality: Jacques Lacan and the école freudienne*, J. Mitchell and J. Rose (eds), trans. J. Rose, New York: Norton, 1982.

Laplanche, J. and Pontalis, J.-B., *The Language of Psycho-Analysis*, trans. D. Nicholson-Smith, New York: Norton, 1973.

Latour, B., *We Have Never Been Modern*, trans. C. Porter, Cambridge, MA: Harvard University Press, 1993.

Lévi-Strauss, C. *The Savage Mind*, Chicago: University of Chicago Press, 1966.

Love, N., *Marx, Nietzsche, and Modernity*, New York: Columbia University Press, 1986.

Lukács, G., *History and Class Consciousness*, trans. R. Livingstone, Cambridge, MA: MIT Press, 1971.

Lyotard, J.-F., *Libidinal Economy*, trans. I. Hamilton Grant, Bloomington: Indiana University Press; London: Athlone Press, 1993.

Macksey, R. and Donato, E. (eds), *The Structuralist Controversy: the Languages of Criticism and the Sciences of Man*, Baltimore, MD: Johns Hopkins University Press, 1972.

Marcuse, H., *Eros and Civilization: a Philosophical Inquiry into Freud*, Boston, MA: Beacon, 1974.

Marx, K., *Capital*, 3 vols, New York: International Publishers, 1967.

—— *Grundrisse: Introduction to the Critique of Political Economy*, trans. M. Nicolaus, New York: Vintage, 1973.

—— *Early Writings*, Q. Hoare (ed.), New York: Vintage, 1975.

—— *On Revolution*, trans. S. Padover, New York: McGraw-Hill, 1971.

Massumi, B., *A User's Guide to Capitalism and Schizophrenia: Deviations from Deleuze and Guattari*, Cambridge, MA: MIT Press, 1992.

Matheron, A., "Le *Traité Théologico-Politique* vu par le jeune Marx," *Cahiers Spinoza*, 1977, vol. 1: 159–212.

Mauss, M., *The Gift*, New York: Norton, 1990.

Merchant, C., *Radical Ecology: the Search for a Liveable World*, New York: Routledge, 1992.

Mitchell, J., *Psychoanalysis and Feminism: Freud, Reich, Laing and Women*, New York: Vintage, 1975.

Mitzman, A., *The Iron Cage: an Historical Interpretation of Max Weber*, New Brunswick: Transaction Books, 1985.

Muller, J. and Richardson, W. (eds.), *The Purloined Poe: Lacan, Derrida, and Psychoanalytic Reading*, Baltimore, MD: Johns Hopkins University Press, 1988.

Negri, A., *Marx Beyond Marx: Lessons on the* Grundrisse, trans. H. Cleaver, M. Ryan, and M. Viano, New York: Bergin & Garvey, 1984.

—— *Revolution Retrieved: Writings on Marx, Keynes, Capitalist Crisis and New Social Subjects, 1967–83*, London: Red Notes, 1988.

—— *The Politics of Subversion: A Manifesto for the Twenty-First Century*, trans. J. Newell, London: Polity Press [Blackwell], 1989.

—— *The Savage Anomaly: the Power of Spinoza's Metaphysics and Politics*, trans. M. Hardt, Minneapolis: University of Minnesota Press, 1991.

Ness, A., *Freedom, Emotion and Self-Subsistence*, Oslo: Universitets-forlaget, 1975.

—— "Spinoza and ecology," in *Speculum Spinozanum, 1677–1977*, S. Hessing (ed.), London: Routledge & Kegan Paul, 1977, 418–25.

Nietzsche, F., *On the Genealogy of Morals*, trans. W. Kaufmann and R. J. Hollingdale, New York: Vintage, 1967.

O'Connor, J., "Capitalism, nature, socialism: a theoretical introduction," in *Capitalism, Nature, Socialism*, 1988, vol. 1: 1–15.

Patton, P. (ed.), *Deleuze: a Critical Reader*, Oxford, and Cambridge, MA: Blackwell, 1996.

Poulantzas, N., *Classes in Contemporary Capitalism*, London: New Left Books, 1975.

Reich, W., *The Function of the Orgasm: Sex-Economic Problems of Biological Energy*, trans. T. P. Wolfe, New York: World Publishing, 1971.

Rubel, M., "Marx à la rencontre de Spinoza," *Cahiers Spinoza*, 1977, vol. 1: 7–28.

Sartre, J.-P., *Critique of Dialectical Reason*, 2 vols, London, and New York: Verso, 1991.

Spinoza, B., *The Ethics and Other Works*, trans. E. Curley, Princeton, NJ: Princeton University Press, 1994.

Sturgeon, N., *Ecofeminist Natures: Race, Gender, Feminist Theory, and Political Action*, New York: Routledge, 1997.

Ulmer, G., *Applied Grammatology*, Baltimore, MD: Johns Hopkins University Press, 1985.

Virilio, P., *Popular Defense and Ecological Struggles*, trans. M. Polizzotti, New York: Semiotext(e), 1990.

Waelhens, A. de., *Schizophrenia: a Philosophical Reflection on Lacan's Structuralist Interpretation*, trans. W. Ver Eecke, Pittsburgh: Duquesne University Press; Atlantic Highlands, NJ: Humanities Press, 1978.

Warren, K. (ed.), *Ecological Feminism*, New York: Routledge, 1994.

—— (ed.), *Ecofeminism: Women, Culture, Nature*, Bloomington: Indiana University Press, 1997.

Weber, M., *The Protestant Ethic and the Spirit of Capitalism*, trans. T. Parsons, New York: Scribner, 1976.

Weeks, K., "Subject for a feminist standpoint," in S. Makdisi, C. Casarino, and R. Karl (eds), *Marxism Beyond Marxism*, New York: Routledge, 1996, 89–118.

Wittgenstein, L., *Philosophical Investigations*, trans. G. E. M. Anscombe, New York: Macmillan, 1953.

Zizek, S., *The Sublime Object of Ideology*, London and New York: Verso, 1989.

—— *For They Know Not What They Do: Enjoyment as a Political Factor*, London and New York: Verso, 1991.

INDEX

accumulation 13, 65–6, 82, 94, 97, 103, 110

Adorno, T. 11–2

alienation 8, 13, 93, 96, 100

alliance 66, 71, 72–7, 79, 83–5, 89, 96–9, 102, 115

Althusser, L. 109–11

ambivalence 12, 38, 57, 61, 89, 92, 94–5, 120–1; *see also* body-without-organs, representation

anti-production 13, 31–4, 36, 57; capitalist 68, 79, 83–4, 96, 112–3; despotic 74–5, 95; and primal repression 57; psychodynamics of 28–9, 96, 115, 122; savage 69–74; social relations of 60–5, 69, 96, 122; *see also* death instinct, expenditure

art 32, 106–7, 123

Artaud, A. 27, 28, 30

asceticism 4, 11, 24, 97, 100, 109, 112, 115; and capitalism 12–13, 64, 85–6, 100–1, 123; and immanent anti-production 83; and the nuclear family 13, 55–6, 60, 84–6, 118–19, 121–3; *see also* Nietzsche

autocritique 15–18, 24, 39, 46, 60, 87, 95–6, 97, 109, 122; *see also* critique, universal history

axiomatization 12, 84–5, 103, 106, 107, 108–9, 116, 121, 123; and coding 64, 66–7, 68, 80, 81–2, 86–7, 91–2, 98, 104, 115; continual expansion of 79–81, 102, 112, 114; and territorialization 20–1, 67–8, 92, 104–5, 120

Bataille, G. 5, 61–3, 112, 114–5; *see also* expenditure

belief 2–3, 12, 21, 35, 39, 48, 52, 60, 63, 66, 67, 80, 83, 85, 87, 94, 98–9; *see also* decoding, paranoia

Bey, H. 108

biosphere 112, 115

body-without-organs 1, 3, 33, 93–4; at end of history 61, 95–7, 120–1, 123; and socius 61, 92, 120–1, 122–3; synthesis of recording on 27–33, 36, 38–9, 96, 57, 93; underlying subjectivity 33–6; *see also* ambivalence

boss 5, 55, 85, 97

Brown, N.O. 8–11

Butler, J. 120–1

capitalism 1, 28, 33, 39, 57, 78, 101, 108, 109; and asceticism 12–13, 24, 95–6, 100–101, 112–13; economics of 15, 19–20, 59–60, 66–8, 78–9, 80–3, 86, 96, 107–8, 113–15; and the family 2, 7, 13, 17–19, 24, 36, 39–41, 44, 49, 52, 55–7, 58–9, 61, 65, 69, 81–2, 83–6, 87–9, 91–3, 105, 118; and gender 116–18, 120–1; and paranoia 2–3, 21, 93, 98–9; and power 59–60, 80–1, 95–6, 98, 122–3; psychodynamics of 3, 7–9, 11, 16–18, 21, 23–4, 83–7, 91, 95–6, 104–6, 112–3, 116–17, 121–2; and schizophrenia 2–3, 21, 54, 59, 65, 93; and the state 78–9, 82; as third socius 58–64, 66–8, 79–80, 87, 92–3, 94, 96–7, 101–2, 112, 114–15, 121–3; and universal history 11, 16–19, 61, 92–3, 94–5, 109–11, 121, 123; *see also*

155

Printed in the United States
by Baker & Taylor Publisher Services

Printed in the United States
by Baker & Taylor Publisher Services